T0327548

Radiology and Follow-up of Urologic Surgery

Radiology and Follow-up of Urologic Surgery

Edited by

Christopher Woodhouse, MB, FRCS, FEBU
University College London, UK

Alex Kirkham, MB BCh, FRCS, FRCR, MD
University College London Hospitals, UK

First Edition

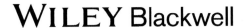

Registered Offices
John Wiley & Sons, Inc., 111 River Street, Hoboken, NJ 07030, USA
John Wiley & Sons Ltd, The Atrium, Southern Gate, Chichester, West Sussex, PO19 8SQ, UK

Editorial Office
9600 Garsington Road, Oxford, OX4 2DQ, UK

For details of our global editorial offices, customer services, and more information about Wiley products visit us at www.wiley.com.

Wiley also publishes its books in a variety of electronic formats and by print-on-demand. Some content that appears in standard print versions of this book may not be available in other formats.

Library of Congress Cataloging-in-Publication Data applied for
9781119162087

Cover Design: Wiley
Cover Image: © 7activestudio/Gettyimages

Set in 10/12pt WarnockPro by SPi Global, Chennai, India

10 9 8 7 6 5 4 3 2 1

Dedicated to our lifelong supporters, Anna Terrington and John Kirkham,
and to our contributors.

Contents

List of Contributors

Clare Allen, BM BCh, FRCR
Consultant Uro-radiologist
University College London Hospital NHS
Trust
London, UK

Christopher Anderson, MB ChB, FCS(Urol)SA, FRCS
Consultant Urologist
Director of Cancer Services
St George's Hospital
London, UK

Daniella E. Andrich, MD, MSc, FRCS(Urol)
Consultant Reconstructive Urologist
University College London Hospital NHS
Trust
London, UK

Bruce Berlanstein, MD
Department of Medicine and Radiology
The Johns Hopkins University School of
Medicine
Baltimore, MA, USA

Simon Bugeja, MD, MRCS(Ed), FEBU, MSc(Urol)
Associate Specialist in Reconstructive
Urology
University College London Hospital NHS
Trust
London, UK

Patrick Dewan, PhD, MD, MS, MMedSc, FRCS, FRACS
Professor of Pediatric Urology and Chairman
Kind Cuts For Kids
Chairman, Wee Kids
Parkville
Victoria, Australia

Alison Elstob, BM BS, MRCS, FRCR
Radiology Fellow
St George's Hospital
London, UK

Mark R. Feneley, MD(Cantab), FRCS(Eng), FRCS(Urol)
Consultant Urologist, University College
London Hospitals
Honorary Senior Lecturer, University
College London
London, UK

Hash Hashim, MB BS, MRCS, MD, FEBU, FRCS(Urol)
Consultant Urological Surgeon and Director
of the Urodynamics Unit
Honorary Senior Lecturer, University of
Bristol
Bristol Urological Institute
Bristol, UK

Richard Hautmann, MD, MD(hon)
Professor of Urology
Chairman Emeritus
Department of Urology
University of Ulm
Neu-Ulm, Germany

Mohamed Ismail, MB ChB, MRCS, FRCS(Urol), PhD
Consultant Urological Surgeon
Portsmouth Hospitals NHS Trust
Queen Alexandra hospital
Portsmouth, UK

Alex Kirkham, MB BCh, FRCS, FRCR, MD
Consultant Radiologist
University College London Hospitals
London, UK

Pardeep Kumar, MB ChB, PhD, FRCS(Urol)
Consultant Urologist
The Royal Marsden Hospital
London, UK

Graham Munneke, MB BS, MRCP, FRCR
Consultant Uro-Radiologist
University College Hospital
London, UK

David Nicol, MB BS, FRACS
Professor of Surgical Oncology
The Institute of Cancer Research
Consultant Urologist and Chief of Surgery
Royal Marsden Hospital
London, UK

Jonathon Olsburgh, MB ChB, FRCS(Urol), PhD
Consultant Transplant and Urological
Surgeon
Guy's and St Thomas' NHS Foundation Trust
London, UK

Doug Pendse, MB ChB, MD, MRCS, FRCR
Consultant Radiologist
University College London Hospitals NHS
Trust
London, UK

Padma Rao, BSc, MB BS, MRCP, FRCR, FRANZCR
Director of Medical Imaging, Royal
Children's Hospital, Melbourne
Honorary Senior Lecturer, University of
Melbourne
Royal Children's Hospital, Melbourne
Parkville, Victoria, Australia

Giles Rottenberg, MB BS, MRCP, FRCR
Consultant Radiologist
Guy's and St Thomas' NHS Foundation Trust
London, UK

Paul J. Scheel, MD, FASN
CEO and Associate Vice Chancellor for
Clinical Affairs
Washington University School of Medicine
St. Louis, MO, USA

Daron Smith, MA(Cantab), BM BCh(Oxon), MD, FRCS(Urol)
Consultant Endoluminal Endourologist
Institute of Urology
University College London Hospital NHS
Trust
London, UK

Aslam Sohaib, MB, MRCP, FRCR
Consultant Radiologist
Royal Marsden Hospital
London, UK

Bjoern G. Volkmer, MD
Professor of Radiology and Head of
Department
Klinikum Kassel
Kassel, Germany

Christopher Woodhouse, MB, FRCS, FEBU
Emeritus Professor of Adolescent Urology
University College London
London, UK

Rhana H. Zakri, MB BS, MRCS, MSc, FRCS(urol)
Specialist Registrar in Transplant & Urology
Guy's and St Thomas' NHS Foundation Trust
London, UK

Acknowledgements

The heroes of this book are the contributing authors. Without exception they found the subject to be intriguing because it had not been tackled before. Then, for the same reason, they found that the lack of evidence-based literature made the writing difficult. All have risen to the challenge, giving the benefit of their experience and analysis of the limited literature. We send them all our greatest thanks.

At Wiley, we have had wonderful support from a most comprehensive team. Walter Oliver, in his last days at the company, pushed hard for the project's acceptance. He was followed by James Schultz and now Deidre Barry who have kept it on track.

Yoga Mohanakrishnan sorted out the submission and established order from multiple files and then Manish Luthra and Shobana Ramesh reviewed the technical aspects of text, images and layout. Dr Laurence Errington has provide a most comprehensive index.

The copy editing was done by Jan East. This is a task that requires meticulous attention to detail and great tact. With her encouragement and gentle pressure everything, down to the smallest detail, was prepared for typesetting on time.

No good book can be produced without such tireless help. We are most grateful to all.

Christopher Woodhouse
Alex Kirkham

Introduction

Christopher Woodhouse and Alex Kirkham

The literature in radiology and urology is predominantly orientated to diagnosis and disease management. Although complications and outcomes are included under 'management', the clinician is often left in the dark about anatomical and physiological changes that follow successful treatment. This is particularly true where there has been conservative or reconstructive surgery. We are faced with patients who have a new set of symptoms, images that look different from those seen before treatment and physiology that requires definition of new normal values.

Clinicians are therefore left wondering what is a complication and what an inevitable consequence of the management? What, for example, is the normal appearance of a kidney cancer after radiofrequency ablation (RFA) and what does a local recurrence look like? How does the urine flow down the ureters after a trans-uretero-ureterostomy? What is the new normal appearance of the urinary tract after a cystoplasty?

When we asked our colleagues to contribute chapters, their reactions were consistent. After the usual complaints of being too busy and so on, there was recognition that the subjects were very intriguing and had not been tackled before. Their instructions emphasised that we were not interested in *why* any particular treatment was carried out, or what the figures for outcome were. We needed the 'new normal' and the differences between that and complications. In some conditions the principal changes were radiological, but biochemical and histological findings also change after some reconstructions. With long-term survival after many reconstructive procedures there are some changes that are the consequence of ageing or the initiation of a malignant change. On the basis of the known changes, what should be the follow-up? This last was often the most difficult because it was rare to find any evidence-based follow-up protocols!

Once our contributors had settled down to their work, all admitted to finding it interesting but challenging. One or two, sadly, felt that the whole task was beyond them. Once completed, however, they universally felt that it had been worthwhile and we, the editors, feel that those who did accept the challenge have triumphed and produced excellent texts and illustrations.

It could be asked why these issues have been so little considered in the literature. Anatomical reconstruction could not begin until it became possible to operate for longer than the few minutes that were needed to chop off a leg or some other damaged appendage, and, even more importantly, to have an aseptic field. The first urological reconstruction of this era was the uretero-sigmoidostomy (U-sig). Simon described this operation in 1852 in a paper in *The Lancet*. If one reads beyond the title it is found that it was a report of an operation that was successful but the patient died. Despite this unhappy beginning, the U-sig

Radiology and Follow-up of Urologic Surgery, First Edition. Edited by Christopher Woodhouse and Alex Kirkham.
© 2018 John Wiley & Sons Ltd. Published 2018 by John Wiley & Sons Ltd.

remained the standard urinary diversion until the ileal conduit was developed in 1948. It had many complications and patients were not always continent, but it usually lasted for 10 years before death occurred from something which, at the time, might have appeared unrelated to the original operation.

In the 100 years during which the U-sig was the predominant lower urinary tract reconstruction, there were plenty of ideas for alternatives. Leon Krynski (1896), a Polish surgeon, described a non-refluxing method of implantation of the ureters into the colon virtually identical to the Politano–Leadbetter procedure. In a textbook published in Leipzig in 1909, Verhoogen and Graeuwe, surgeons from Brussels, reviewed the possibilities of continent diversions. They quoted Pawlik (1889) who created a new bladder by diverting the urine into the vagina; continence was achieved by tightening of the introitus and the patient was continent and could void. Verhoogen had made a reservoir from the caecum and drained to skin by the appendix. The accompanying diagram (Figure I.1) showed a system very similar to that used today. The results were not recorded.

Clean intermittent catheterisation (CIC) was described by Lapides *et al.* in 1972. It is interesting to note that none of the early reports of bladder reconstructions described how the reservoir was to be emptied. There are anecdotal reports of men keeping catheters in their hat bands, which could be described as dirty self-catheterisation!

In this phase of anatomical reconstruction, Anderson and Hynes (1949) described their procedure for anastomosing the retro-caval ureter to the renal pelvis. This was not then carried out to treat pelvi-ureteric obstruction although it is now. Trendelenberg (1906) designed a bladder reconstruction for exstrophy which allowed the paediatric patient to void, albeit only for a short time before the wound broke open. Dennis-Brown (1936) described his 'buried skin strip' operation for hypospadias which has some similarity to the current Snodgrass procedure. It should

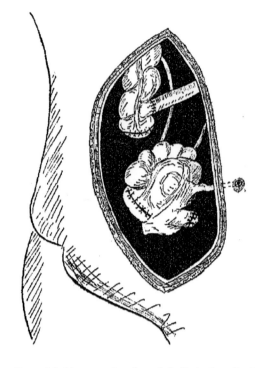

Figure I.1 Diagram taken from *Folio Urologica* edited by James Israel, Leipzig, 1909, pp. 629–679. It shows the construction of a urinary reservoir from caecum and drained by the appendix, attributed to Verhoogan. With thanks to Professor Elmar Gerharz who first drew our attention to this fascinating book.

be noted that at least 51 'new' operations for hypospadias were described in the twentieth century. Sadove *et al.* (1993) used a vascularised graft of fibula and overlying soft tissue to replace the small or absent penis.

Despite all of these ideas and clinical experiments, it is really only since the 1980s that reconstructive urology has become a major subspecialty and produced the large numbers of long-term survivors from single institutions that are needed for study.

The other criterion for inclusion in this book is 'conservative surgery'. Conservation as a surgical concept generally implies greater difficulty with preservation of blood and nerve supply. At least until the 1960s, cancer was generally treated by radical surgery or radiotherapy, partly because it was known that malignant cells could be found outside the visible mass and partly because there was no other treatment. Later it was recognised that less radical surgery, sometimes augmented by radiotherapy (or, later, chemotherapy), could achieve the same result with less morbidity. Now, conservative surgery is often supplemented by reconstruction and performed with minimal access technology.

There are the same issues with follow-up as there are with reconstructive surgery: what does the conserved organ look like; how does it work; what is a complication and what does a malignant recurrence look like?

The book has a section for each of the organs of the genitourinary tract and the chapters are based on the major diseases and operations that are used. There are copious illustrations, a feature strongly encouraged by the excellent staff at Wiley Blackwell. We are very aware of the difficulties that the contributors have had and the time that they have devoted to their work. We are most grateful to them all and especially for the new light that they have shone on the outcomes of urological surgery beyond the standard survival and complication rates.

1

Subtotal Nephrectomy and Tumour Ablation

David Nicol, Alison Elstob, Christopher Anderson and Graham Munneke

Introduction

With the use of cross-sectional imaging, small renal tumours have been increasingly diagnosed over the past 20 years [1]. During this period, management has become more conservative with a progressive decline in the utilisation of radical nephrectomy. Nephron-sparing approaches have been widely adopted with the objectives of preserving renal function and reducing long-term morbidity. Partial nephrectomy with excision or enucleation of the tumour appears to have equivalent oncological outcomes to more radical surgery. The availability of robotically assisted surgery allows a minimally invasive procedure for partial nephrectomy that many now suggest is the surgical procedure of choice when feasible. Ablative therapies such as radiofrequency ablation (RFA) and cryoablation (CA) are alternatives to partial and radical nephrectomy, particularly for patients who are not suitable surgical candidates. Small renal masses in the short to intermediate term frequently exhibit slow growth and minimal metastatic risk and consequently surveillance is now adopted in patients who are elderly or have significant co-morbidities.

Postoperative and follow-up imaging after radical nephrectomy for small renal tumours is essentially to detect early postoperative complications and the relatively rare events of local recurrence and metastatic disease.

The increasingly utilised nephron-sparing approaches have introduced challenges associated with the repeated imaging that is required for these various options. These include investigations of the tumour-bearing kidney for a range of specific complications of the various strategies as well as the possibility of incomplete eradication, tumour recurrence within the remaining parenchyma as well as disease progression. Anatomical distortion of the kidney and evolving changes to masses subjected to ablative treatment or undergoing surveillance management represent specific challenges for the nephron-sparing approaches.

Procedures

Partial Nephrectomy

Surgical excision of small renal tumours is undertaken as either an open operation or, increasingly, with a robotically assisted or laparoscopic approach. Tumours can be enucleated or excised with a margin of surrounding renal parenchyma. Components of the operation include mobilisation of the kidney and identification of the renal mass, isolation of the renal artery, with temporary occlusion/clamping if required, tumour excision and renal repair. The last may, in some cases, require closure of the collecting system in addition to oversewing of the incised parenchyma including divided blood

Radiology and Follow-up of Urologic Surgery, First Edition. Edited by Christopher Woodhouse and Alex Kirkham.
© 2018 John Wiley & Sons Ltd. Published 2018 by John Wiley & Sons Ltd.

vessels required for haemostasis. A ureteric stent can be inserted as a preliminary or during surgery if collecting system repair is required.

Follow-up imaging is required to assess and guide management of early postoperative complications, most often haemorrhage or urinary leakage. Longer term imaging is also required as routine to detect local recurrence either at the site of resection or within the remaining parenchyma.

Early Imaging

This is principally indicated for assessment of clinically recognised or suspected complications of the surgical procedure and to direct their management. Haemorrhage and urinary leakage comprise the principal surgical complications that require imaging.

Haemorrhage Bleeding can arise in the initial postoperative period, usually reflecting an unsecured artery, or days to weeks later as a result of rupture of a pseudo-aneurysm of an intrarenal artery. The events alerting the clinician are signs of blood loss or falling haematocrit as well as flank pain or mass and at times, heavy haematuria. Subtle unexplained drops in haematocrit, which may precede signs of significant bleeding, can also prompt radiological investigation. The principal investigations used are computerised tomographic angiography (CTA) and invasive angiography [2].

CTA – may be required initially to determine the source of blood loss. Intravenous contrast should be employed as this will assist localisation of bleeding. Recommended imaging entails an initial arterial phase after bolus contrast injection with a subsequent portal venous phase approximately 1 minute later [3]. Visualisation of active bleeding based on contrast extravasation is an indication for urgent embolisation (Figure 1.1). Whether CTA is a necessary preliminary to standard angiography, required for embolisation, is debatable. In the context of bleeding following partial nephrectomy from the kidney, CTA may be a redundant investigation increasing contrast media exposure as angiography and embolisation is highly likely to be required. When CTA fails to detect an active source, angiography may also be deemed necessary based on clinical concern and heightened suspicion. In practice it is often used as a rapidly accessible investigation and to confirm whether bleeding is from the kidney itself, from non-renal vessels such as lumbar or intercostal or reflects damage to other organs such as the spleen or liver which may not be evident on selective angiography.

In cases where there are significant concerns regarding contrast and specifically renal dysfunction, ultrasound (US) and magnetic resonance angiography (MRA) are alternative options. Of these, MRA, if available, is the best alternative to CTA in providing detail of the intrarenal circulation

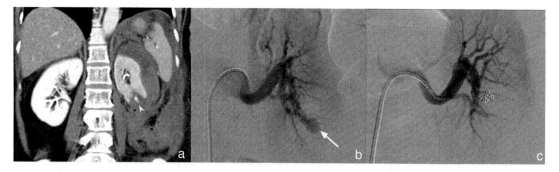

Figure 1.1 Haemorrhage 7 days following left partial nephrectomy with large perinephric haematoma and contrast extravasation on computerised tomography (CT) (a). On subsequent angiography, no sign of active bleeding persisted but a contained lower pole aneurysm was demonstrated (arrow, b) which was successfully treated with gel embolisation (c).

as well as assessment of non-renal bleeding sources. US can exclude other bleeding sites, such as the liver or spleen, but apart from this and the presence of a perinephric haematoma provides little additional information. Therefore its use may be of little value if there is clinical evidence of bleeding.

Angiography is used both diagnostically and for selective embolisation as the preferred management of the bleeding source [4]. To minimise contrast exposure, this is performed selectively with initial study of the renal artery to localise the source of bleeding. This may demonstrate an obvious pseudo-aneurysm or outline extravasation of contrast from an involved vessel. Manipulation of the angiographic catheter into the involved vessel is then undertaken, with coils being deployed to occlude the lumen and control bleeding. Multiple coils may be required to achieve occlusion and on occasions repeat procedures are required – as intrarenal vasospasm may masquerade as adequate control with subsequent further bleeding. Whilst super selective embolisation is preferred, this may not prove feasible or successful. In this circumstance, larger vessels may need to be occluded resulting in loss of some of the remaining renal parenchyma.

Urinary Leakage Urinary leakage arises from either the collecting system or the ureter or renal pelvis if these were damaged at the time of the procedure [5]. These problems present as urine leakage from a drain, renal dysfunction or flank mass/pain in the absence of bleeding. US may demonstrate a fluid collection around the kidney prompting formal assessment with a CT urogram (Figure 1.2). This will confirm the presence of urinoma and outline the site and nature of leakage with extravasation of contrast from the collecting system or ureter. Hydronephrosis may also be seen on US and CT – which may relate to distal obstruction resulting from luminal clot, ureteric compression by the urinoma or a consequence of ureteric injury.

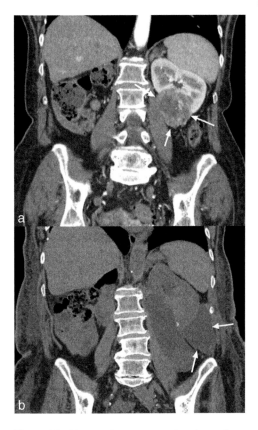

Figure 1.2 A large urinoma presenting 4 months after a partial nephrectomy. The arrows in (a) show the tumour. A ureteric stent was placed at time of surgery in view of the major collecting system repair. The stent had been removed electively 4 weeks prior to representation with left flank discomfort; the urinoma is shown by the arrows in (b).

Late Imaging

Tumour recurrence is the principal goal of longer term imaging. Currently, there are no standardised guidelines regarding the preferred imaging modality or the frequency with which it should be performed. US, CT and magnetic resonance imaging (MRI) are all used. Anatomical and functional changes can also be seen in the course of planned follow-up imaging.

Anatomical Changes Distortion of the renal parenchyma may complicate the interpretation of studies. Imaging is thus recommended 3–6 months following surgery to redefine the anatomical appearances of the kidney as a baseline for longer term follow-up. A resection defect will usually be apparent, reflecting the excised segment of kidney – often more complex if the initial tumour was central or hilar.

Techniques used to secure haemostasis and close the excision defect can also confound the interpretation of imaging [6]. These include portions of revascularised perinephric fat (Figure 1.3) and haemostatic agents (e.g. oxidised cellulose; Figure 1.4) [7]. Inflammatory reactions including foreign body granulomas reported with the latter may result in pseudo-tumour formation resulting in a diagnostic dilemma [8]. With surveillance, these remain stable or gradually involute although complete regression may not occur. Similar reactions have been reported with other biomaterials used to secure haemostasis [8]. Perinephric haematomas or urine collection at the site of resection can also result in abscess formation (Figures 1.5 and 1.6) and

can develop weeks to months following surgery [7].

Haematomas and small urinomas at the site of resection can also create effects that may masquerade as recurrent disease. These may appear complex with solid and cystic elements as a consequence of inflammation and clot organisation. These may be evident on imaging at 3–6 months but resolve gradually over time (Figure 1.7).

Functional Changes The following types of late complications can be observed as a consequence of surgery:

- *Vascular* Renal artery pseudo-aneurysm may present asymptomatically as an incidental finding as a complex vascularised mass (Figure 1.8). Systematic radiological evaluation suggests that these occur in up to 20% of cases during the early postoperative period after partial nephrectomy [2]. They usually resolve spontaneously but may leave a persistent residual mass which may be difficult to distinguish from recurrent disease [9].

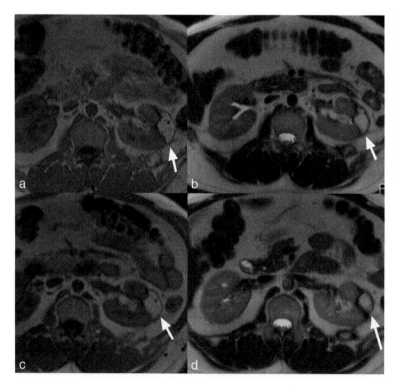

Figure 1.3 Magnetic resonance imaging (MRI) of a patient who underwent left partial nephrectomy with placement of perinephric fat into the defect (arrow) at 3 months on (a) T1 and (b) T2 axial images. (c,d) T1 and T2 images at 15 months. No changes were observed over this time.

Figure 1.4 Contrast-enhanced CT: (a) 3 months after partial nephrectomy demonstrating a lesion with a hypodense non-enhancing outer portion where oxidised cellulose had been placed and an inner isodense enhancing area representing granuloma formation; (b) T2 MRI showing hypointense outer and hyperintense inner; and (c) contrast-enhanced MRI showing enhancement only in the inner portion.

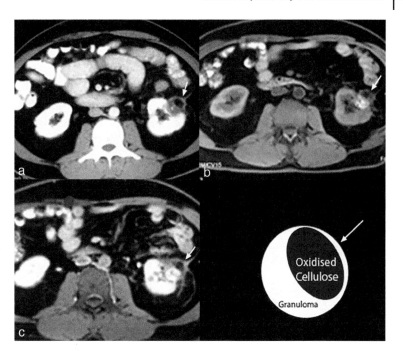

Figure 1.5 (a) Axial and (b) coronal CT images demonstrated a rim enhancing collection (arrow) containing locules of gas at the site of recent partial nephrectomy. (c) The abscess was managed with CT-guided drainage. (d) The drain was subsequently up-sized under fluoroscopic guidance to ensure complete drainage.

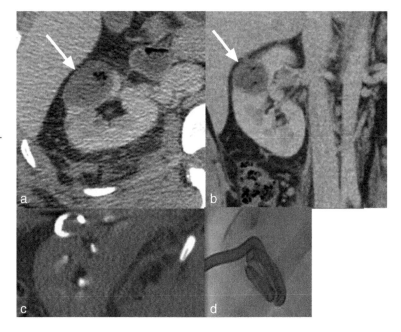

- *Ischaemia* Ischaemic injury can occur to the kidney reflecting parenchymal effects of prolonged renal artery clamping. Renal ischaemia can also evolve from the effects of renal artery manipulation. Thrombosis of the renal artery may occur in the postoperative period with complete infarction of the kidney which subsequently undergoes global atrophy. Renal artery stenosis can also occur although this may be

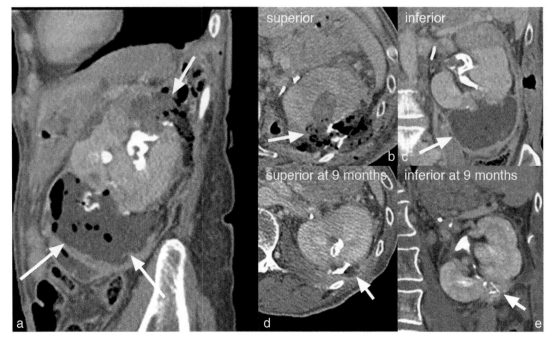

Figure 1.6 Following a two-site left partial nephrectomy: (a) sagittal CT imaging demonstrated two discrete enhancing collections (superior b, inferior c) consistent with infected urinomas. (d,e) Interval CT imaging at 9 months following percutaneous drainage and decompression with retrograde stenting showed resolution.

difficult to distinguish from the effects of intraoperative ischaemia. Severe hypertension prompts angiographic assessment and consideration of renal vein renin sampling.

- *Obstruction* Ureteric stenosis can result in proximal ureteric and collecting system dilatation, reflecting direct ureteric injury or ischaemia as a result of cautery or other trauma to its blood supply if aggressively mobilised or retracted during the surgical event (Figure 1.9). Intrarenal obstruction to one or more calyces may also arise insidiously, reflecting infundibular damage related to ischaemia or an effect of collecting system repair or closure of the parenchymal defect.

Recurrent Tumour Tumour recurrence occurs in a small proportion of cases following partial nephrectomy [10]. This may occur at the margins of the resection and reflects either incomplete excision or a separate satellite lesion that has progressed. Further tumours may also occur remotely within the remaining parenchyma, with patients with hereditary disorders at highest risk. From the imaging point of view they have the same characteristics as the original tumour.

Ablative Therapies

Image-guided ablation with use of thermal energy is now frequently used as an alternative to surgical excision of small renal tumours. The currently employed modalities are RFA and CA [11]. RFA results in coagulation of tissue as radiofrequency waves delivered continuously via a probe are converted to heat producing thermal tissue damage. In contrast, CA involves rapid freeze–thaw cycles delivered through probes inserted into the tumour producing ice formation and disrupting cellular membranes resulting in tissue necrosis and injury to local microvasculature. The volume of treatment has to be slightly larger than the tumour area to ensure adequate ablation.

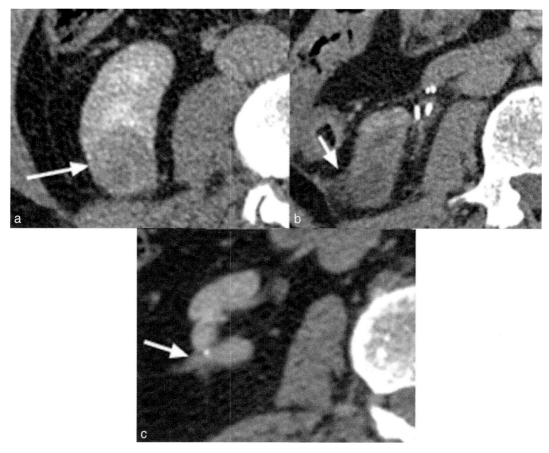

Figure 1.7 (a) Right lower pole tumour at presentation. (b) At 6 months post partial nephrectomy. (c) At 6 years post partial nephrectomy.

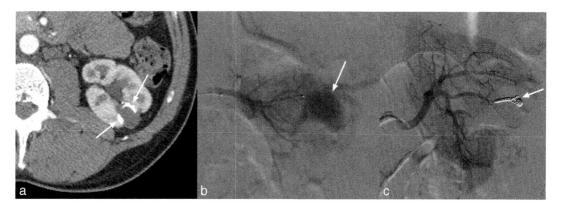

Figure 1.8 Asymptomatic pseudo-aneurysm identified 18 months after partial nephrectomy. Curvilinear calcification seen on CT (arrows, a) with pseudo-aneurysm demonstrated on angiography (b). This was treated with coil embolisation (c).

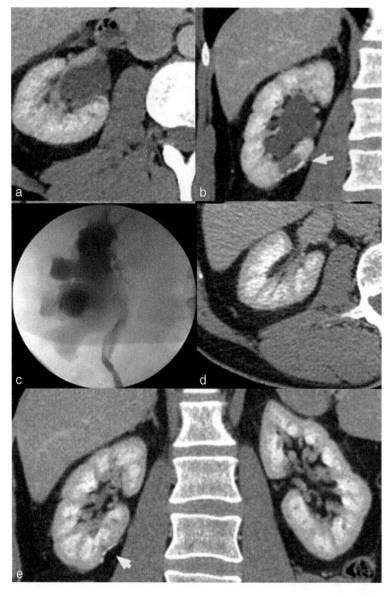

Figure 1.9 (a) Axial and (b) coronal CT images demonstrated new hydronephrosis at 6 months post partial nephrectomy for a right lower pole lesion. (c) Retrograde pyelogram obtained at the time of retrograde dilatation and stenting. (d,e) Subsequent CT at 12 months demonstrated resolution of the hydronephrosis without further intervention. Non-absorbable polymer sutures (arrows) used to secure haemostasis are seen on (b) and (e).

Whilst there are variations in technical issues, neither modality is clearly superior and preference is largely based on institutional facilities and clinician experience [11]. Currently, both are delivered as CT-guided techniques using a percutaneous approach, although some centres continue to use a laparoscopically guided approach with CA in selected cases.

As the tumour remains in situ following ablative therapies it is imperative that radiological surveillance with cross-sectional imaging is undertaken to exclude residual or recurrent malignancy. There is no consensus regarding frequency or duration of imaging studies [12]. Both MRI and CT can be used and require contrast studies to assess for incomplete ablation and recurrent tumour formation. As the radiological appearances of ablative therapies may evolve over time, serial studies are critical to determine successful treatment. Interpretation of changes

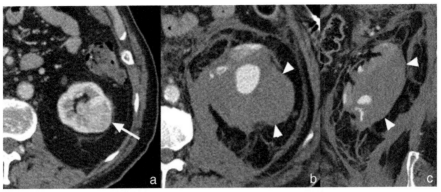

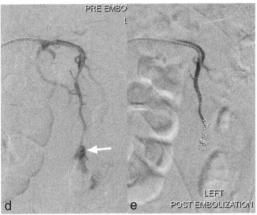

Figure 1.10 Enhancing endophytic renal mass pre-cryoablation (arrow, a). (b) Axial and (c) sagittal post contrast CT images demonstrate acute haemorrhage (arrowheads) at 6 hours post cryoablation. (d) Subsequent angiogram demonstrates acute extravasation from a lower pole segmental artery. (e) Haemostasis was achieved following successful super selective embolisation with micro coils.

to the treated and surrounding areas creates challenges in addition to the long-term burden of follow-up imaging.

Complications

Early Complications Despite its minimally invasive nature both RFA and CA are associated with complications requiring imaging in the early period following the procedure. Some degree of haemorrhage is an expected outcome following percutaneous ablation. If contrast is administered immediately after CA bleeding may be seen along the applicator tracts [13]. Most scans during or immediately following renal ablation procedures will show some evidence of perinephric haematoma, regardless of the technology used [13]. Whilst the vast majority are subclinical, significant haemorrhage can occur and may be both perinephric (Figure 1.10) and subcapsular (Figure 1.11) [14]. Collecting system and ureteric damage can occur when these structures are adjacent to the treated lesion, resulting in urinoma formation and obstruction [13].

Late Complications As with partial nephrectomy, both RFA and CA may be associated with late complications which may be demonstrated on imaging performed for clinical indications or become apparent with follow-up surveillance studies. Subcapsular haematoma may also occur insidiously with compromise to renal function [14]. Ureteric

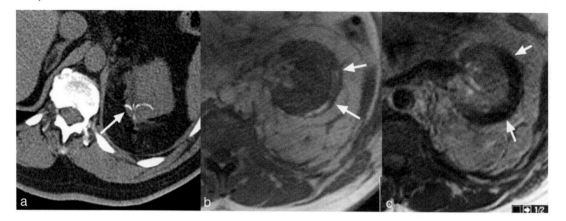

Figure 1.11 Following radiofrequency ablation (RFA) for an upper pole renal mass measuring 3 cm (arrow, a), a patient represented at 4 days with persistent left flank pain related to subcapsular haematoma (arrows), seen on (b) T1 and (c) T2-weighted MRI.

stenosis may also be seen on follow-up imaging – typically associated with treatment of medial lower pole masses.

Successful Tumour Ablation

With successful ablation, renal tumours will ultimately appear as focal lesions with no evidence of contrast enhancement on MRI (Figure 1.12) and CT [15]. Whilst there may be a zone of ablation, which can increase in the days following treatment, involution and residual scar formation subsequently occurs if tumour eradication has been successful (Figure 1.13). This can be a relatively slow process, with 30% reduction in the first 6 months. By 3 years the ablation zone size has decreased by an average of 75%. At this point only 40% of cases have undetectable treatment zones on CT or MRI [15]. Consequently, lack of involution of the treated zone is not indicative of treatment failure.

On CT scanning, the treated areas appear as low attenuation regions following both RFA and CA. On MRI, tumours appear isointense to hyperintense on T1-weighted images and hypointense on T2-weighted MRI compared with normal renal parenchyma [15]. Within the treated tumours, necrotic debris and areas of haemorrhage may demonstrate

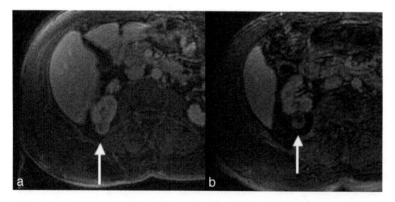

Figure 1.12 Contrast-enhanced T1-weighted MRI (a) before treatment with the renal tumour seen as an avidly enhancing exophytic mass arising from the posterior aspect of the right kidney and (b) immediately following successful radiofrequency ablation where the lesion is now devascularised and does not enhance post contrast.

Figure 1.13 Progressive involution following cryoablation. (a) CT image of a 2.0-cm tumour with changes: (b) at 3 months, (c) 1 year and (d) 2 years following treatment.

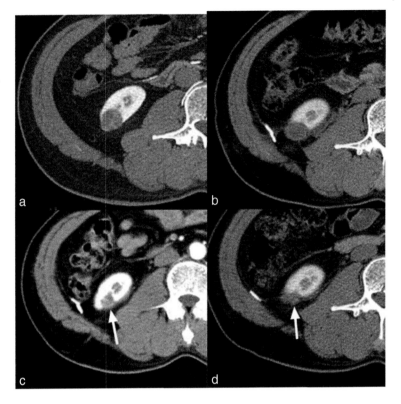

increased signal intensity on MRI. On CT, these appear as areas of increased attenuation. These changes are most apparent during the first few months following treatment.

Following ablative therapies a thin rim of enhancement peripheral to the treated parenchyma can be seen on CT and MRI. This periablational enhancement reflects the physiological response to tissue injury comprising early reactive hyperaemia with subsequent inflammatory cell response and fibrosis [12]. The enhancing component gradually resolves and is often barely visible after 3–6 months. An area or halo of curvilinear hyperattentuation, however, may persist to some extent for years after treatment (Figure 1.14). This benign process appears as an essentially concentric, symmetric and largely uniform process. Its smooth margins need to be distinguished from the irregular peripheral enhancement associated with residual tumour.

Treatment Failure

Contrast enhancement within ablated lesions is generally indicative of the presence of residual tumour. This is typically seen as a nodular (Figure 1.15) or crescentic region peripherally located within the ablated lesion (Figure 1.16). The latter needs to be differentiated from the thin peripheral rim of enhancement that can persist for several months following successful ablation.

Failure of ablative therapy must be suspected with tumour, or parts thereof, that demonstrate increased post-contrast signal intensity on MRI or enhances more than 10 HU with contrast-enhanced CT imaging [12, 15]. Similarly, serial increase in tumour size following treatment should be regarded with suspicion.

Both RFA and CA result in a spherical treatment effect and thus residual tumour generally manifests as enhancing tissue that is nodular or crescentic in shape at the periphery of the ablated tumour. Within

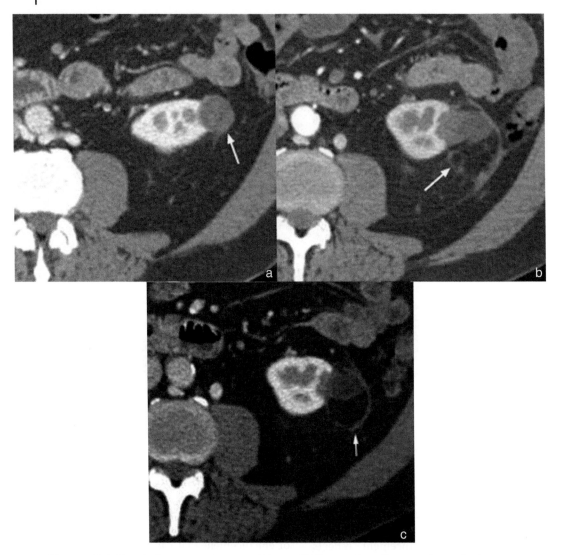

Figure 1.14 (a) Exophytic tumour prior to cryoablation. (b) Venous phase CT scan at 3 months demonstrates a heterogeneous hypodense area in the ablation zone with a curvilinear hyperattentuation area, or 'halo'. (c) At 12 months, ablated lesion shows non-enhancement but persistence of the curvilinear hyperattentuation in the surrounding perinephric fat.

treated lesions, haemorrhage or calcification can produce relatively high attenuation on CT which obviously do not enhance (Figure 1.17). With MRI, subtraction or quantitative assessment is used to assess contrast enhancement, as high signal intensity on T1 images in treated tumours.

Residual hypervascular tumours show avid enhancement with late arterial phase images. Less vascular tumours may demonstrate more delayed contrast enhancement requiring delayed venous images to appreciate [12]. At times, findings may be subtle or equivocal in nature and may prompt early repeat CT or MRI and possible consideration of biopsy – although sampling error may limit its utility [16].

Unfortunately, with ablative therapies residual microscopic foci of tumour may not be identified with current imaging

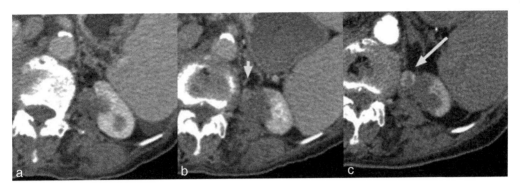

Figure 1.15 Contrast-enhanced axial CT images post percutaneous cryotherapy at 24 months demonstrated a new enhancing 9-mm nodule (arrow, b) in comparison with the 12-month post-treatment scan (a). The nodule demonstrated further growth to 12 mm on the 27-month CT (arrow, c).

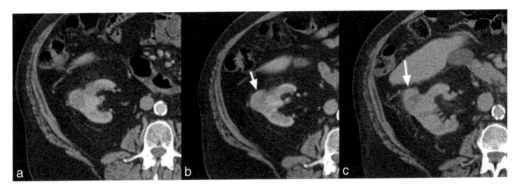

Figure 1.16 Patient who underwent RFA to a 3-cm right renal lesion initially had a favourable CT response at 3 months (a) but on subsequent imaging 6 months later demonstrated enhancing soft tissue nodularity in the periphery of the lesion (arrow, b). This progressed further over a 6-month period with clear tumour recurrence in the anterior aspect of the lesion (c), arrow.

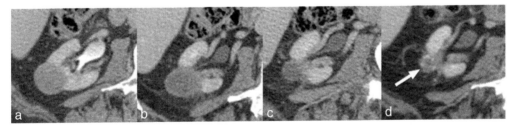

Figure 1.17 (a) An enhancing right renal lesion was treated with percutaneous cryoablation. (b) At 3 months post cryoablation, the lesion no longer demonstrated significant post-contrast enhancement. (c) At 18 months, the lesion had reduced in attenuation and in size. (d) At 4 years, the treated lesion had reduced further in size and was non-enhancing containing areas of peripheral calcification (arrowed) as well as a surrounding halo.

techniques and, consequently, even with apparent radiological success, long-term surveillance imaging is required.

Treatment failure may only become radiologically apparent over time reflecting progression of viable elements of the tumour. Enlargement or subsequent appearance of enhancement within the ablated region following an initially favourable radiological response should be regarded with a high level of suspicion and either closely monitored or considered for investigation and treatment [16].

Surveillance

Small renal tumours are often detected in elderly patients with significant co-morbidities. Many of these tumours have a lower malignant potential, with 20% or more, in fact, being benign lesions such as oncocytomas. Based on series reports, active surveillance (AS) of small renal tumours may be appropriate in elderly patients and even younger patients with co-morbidities. Data from retrospective studies demonstrate that the growth rate for these tumours is slow, with very few progressing to metastatic disease [17]. Consequently, AS with treatment only with evidence of progression is now increasingly practised and is the initial strategy in up to 10% of patients presenting with small renal masses [18]. Radiological studies, employing one or more of US, CT or MRI, do not reliably distinguish between benign and malignant masses <4 cm in diameter. Tumour growth, features or multifocality do not appear particularly useful. An analysis of multiple retrospective AS series suggested only lesions that demonstrated growth developed metastases, with the obvious uncertainty that intervention at presentation would have prevented this [19].

Thus, whilst growth rate of small renal tumours may be a predictor of aggressive disease, this has not been validated in a controlled or prospective fashion. Studies use a range of modalities to assess lesions, with a broad range of clinicians assessing potential changes. Linear dimensions based on diameter is the principal technique used for measuring and reporting tumour size and growth in studies and is the standard in clinical practice. Whilst this is the easiest and most reproducible mechanism to assess and follow masses, it may not be as representative of clinical significance as volumetric assessment – although the latter is not yet a widely used tool.

Follow-up Imaging

Nephron-sparing approaches to renal tumours introduce a requirement for follow-up imaging significantly greater than with nephrectomy. All guidelines, even following nephrectomy, have been generated from retrospective series without prospective evaluation either oncologically or financially [20]. Nor surprisingly, whilst imaging following nephron-sparing approaches is the topic of many publications, there is no consensus or evidence-based guidelines with respect to frequency, duration or modality of imaging [21].

Surveillance studies have highlighted the slow growth of small renal masses, and consequently local recurrence may take considerable time to be radiologically apparent. Follow-up imaging therefore would appear a necessary requirement for nephron-sparing approaches to small renal masses unless final histology has confirmed a benign lesion such as an oncocytoma. Cost considerations and avoidance of repeated contrast exposure would favour the use of US where feasible in the longer term, reserving MRI and CT for when size or features change. As tumour recurrence may have subtle features, which may be slow to become apparent, imaging should always be performed with access to prior studies to characterise accurately the features of any abnormality as well as size of residual lesions over time.

Partial Nephrectomy

Cross-sectional imaging, with either CT or MRI, as well as a US examination of the kidneys at 3–6 months following surgery would seem a sensible approach. This is fundamentally to establish a baseline to enable interpretation of longer term studies and identify unrecognised complications of surgery. With this any changes seen can be reasonably attributed to the procedure as recurrence, particularly in the absence of positive surgical margins, at this time point is extremely unlikely. Subsequent imaging can comprise annual US alone, provided it is a technically satisfactory evaluation, to minimise cost and radiation exposure. Patients with positive surgical margins, larger size (pT1b), adverse histological features, hereditary and multifocal tumours may also warrant more frequent imaging including contrast studies because of heightened concerns regarding local recurrence.

Ablative Therapies

Follow-up imaging is more burdensome with both RFA and CA as residual lesions can remain after apparently successful ablation. The complex features of the residual mass that frequently remains requires contrast-enhanced evaluation to verify treatment success. As with partial nephrectomy, baseline imaging with CT or MRI should be undertaken at 3 months. The intervals between subsequent studies will be dependent on findings, particularly if the ablated mass demonstrates any suspicious features. With complete resolution of the mass or a stable residuum/scar without contrast enhancement, US examination could be substituted after several years to reduce both the cost and other implications of contrast-based studies. This should be continued as recurrence can occur after even complete resolution of a post-treatment mass (Figure 1.18).

Surveillance

To date, there are no consistent criteria for either consideration of AS or follow-up imaging. Clinical judgement and patient preference favour this in selected cases where age or co-morbidities are relevant factors [22]. With solid lesions there is little need for follow-up imaging to be dictated by the need to characterise the mass as the essential trigger for intervention is size. When technically feasible, US is quite adequate to provide linear measurements in several axes. Frequency of imaging is also undetermined although initial reassessments at 3–6 month intervals may be useful for clinician and patient reassurance. Frequency can be reduced if stability of the mass is demonstrated and both the clinician and patient remain comfortable. Complex cystic lesions are more problematic and may require more detailed characterisation with contrast studies [23].

Conclusions

The increased utilisation of nephron-sparing approaches in the management of small renal masses has increased the need for follow-up imaging compared with nephrectomy. The interpretation of radiological findings has also become more challenging.

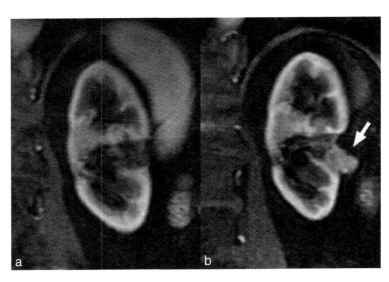

Figure 1.18 (a) No residual abnormality demonstrated at the site of laparoscopic cryotherapy at 3 years post treatment. (b) Further MRI at 4 years post treatment demonstrated an enhancing 2.3-cm mass in the mid pole of the left kidney consistent with recurrence. This was subsequently treated with percutaneous cryotherapy.

This relates to the complications and local effects of treatment as well as the risks of local recurrence and tumour progression. Serial imaging studies are frequently required which may need to be tailored to the individual patient and circumstance. It is also critical that urologists and radiologists work closely in interpreting images in longitudinal sequence because of the evolutionary nature of the changes that may occur.

References

1 Ha SC, Zlomke HA, Cost N, Wilson S. The past, present, and future in management of small renal masses. *J Oncol.* 2015; 2015: 364807.

2 Takagi T, Kondo T, Tajima T, Campbell SC, Tanabe K. Enhanced computed tomography after partial nephrectomy in early postoperative period to detect asymptomatic renal artery pseudoaneurysm. *Int J Urol.* 2014; 21(9): 880–885.

3 Kriegmair MC, Mandel P, Rathmann N, Diehl SJ, Pfalzgraf D, Ritter M. Open partial nephrectomy for high-risk renal masses is associated with renal pseudoaneurysms: assessment of a severe procedure-related complication. *Biomed Res Int.* 2015; 2015: 981251.

4 Tinto HR, Di Primio M, Tselikas L, *et al.* Selective arterial embolization of life-threatening renal hemorrhage in four patients after partial nephrectomy. *Diagn Interv Imaging.* 2014; 95(6): 601–609.

5 Tanagho YS, Kaouk JH, Allaf ME, *et al.* Perioperative complications of robot-assisted partial nephrectomy: analysis of 886 patients at 5 United States centers. *Urology.* 2013; 81(3): 573–579.

6 Pai D, Willatt JM, Korobkin M, *et al.* CT appearances following laparoscopic partial nephrectomy for renal cell carcinoma using a rolled cellulose bolster. *Cancer Imaging.* 2010; 10: 161–168.

7 Lall CG, Patel HP, Fujimoto S, Sandhu S, Sundaram C, Landman J. Making sense of postoperative CT imaging following laparoscopic partial nephrectomy. *Clin Radiol.* 2012; 67(7): 675–686.

8 Agarwal MM, Mandal AK, Agarwal S, *et al.* Surgicel granuloma: unusual cause of 'recurrent' mass lesion after laparoscopic nephron-sparing surgery for renal cell carcinoma. *Urology.* 2010; 76(2): 334–335.

9 Albani JM, Novick AC. Renal artery pseudoaneurysm after partial nephrectomy: three case reports and a literature review. *Urology.* 2003; 62(2): 227–231.

10 Antic T, Taxy JB. Partial nephrectomy for renal tumors: lack of correlation between margin status and local recurrence. *Am J Clin Pathol.* 2015; 143(5): 645–651.

11 Martin J, Athreya S. Meta-analysis of cryoablation versus microwave ablation for small renal masses: is there a difference in outcome? *Diagn Interv Radiol.* 2013; 19(6): 501–507.

12 Iannuccilli JD, Grand DJ, Dupuy DE, Mayo-Smith WW. Percutaneous ablation for small renal masses-imaging follow-up. *Semin Intervent Radiol.* 2014; 31(1): 50–63.

13 Kurup AN. Percutaneous ablation for small renal masses-complications. *Semin Intervent Radiol.* 2014; 31(1): 42–49.

14 Zhao LC, Chan SW, Macejko AM, Lin WW. Percutaneous radiofrequency ablation-induced perinephric hematoma with acute renal failure in a solitary kidney. *J Endourol.* 2008; 22(7): 1463–1465.

15 Kawamoto S, Solomon SB, Bluemke DA, Fishman EK. Computed tomography and magnetic resonance imaging appearance of renal neoplasms after radiofrequency ablation and cryoablation. *Semin Ultrasound CT MR.* 2009; 30(2): 67–77.

16 Breda A, Anterasian C, Belldegrun A. Management and outcomes of tumor recurrence after focal ablation

renal therapy. *J Endourol.* 2010; 24(5): 749–752.

17 Lane BR, Tobert CM, Riedinger CB. Growth kinetics and active surveillance for small renal masses. *Curr Opin Urol.* 2012; 22(5): 353–359.

18 Huang WC, Atoria CL, Bjurlin M, *et al.* Management of small kidney cancers in the new millennium: contemporary trends and outcomes in a population-based cohort. *JAMA Surg.* 2015; 150(7): 664–672.

19 Smaldone MC, Kutikov A, Egleston BL, *et al.* Small renal masses progressing to metastases under active surveillance: a systematic review and pooled analysis. *Cancer.* 2012; 118(4): 997–1006.

20 Kim EH, Strope SA. Postoperative surveillance imaging for patients undergoing nephrectomy for renal cell carcinoma. *Urol Oncol.* 2015; 33(12): 499–502.

21 Ljungberg B, Bensalah K, Canfield S, *et al.* EAU guidelines on renal cell carcinoma: 2014 update. *Eur Urol.* 2015; 67(5): 913–924.

22 Campbell SC, Novick AC, Belldegrun A, *et al.* Guideline for management of the clinical T1 renal mass. *J Urol.* 2009; 182(4): 1271–1279.

23 Ellimoottil C, Greco KA, Hart S, *et al.* New modalities for evaluation and surveillance of complex renal cysts. *J Urol.* 2014; 192(6): 1604–1611.

2

Renal Transplantation

Rhana H. Zakri, Giles Rottenberg and Jonathon Olsburgh

Introduction

The last 61 years of renal transplantation have seen many surgical and medical advances, not least pushing the boundaries with extended criteria for kidney donors and, more recently, minimal access transplant surgery. Complications after renal transplantation are therefore not only varied, but also vast. Discussing all would be beyond the scope of this chapter so we concentrate on commonly encountered surgical (vascular and urological) complications in adult transplant recipients.

To understand transplant complications better, it is pertinent to highlight how a normal kidney transplant appears on ultrasound (US).

The Role of Ultrasound Imaging

Greyscale and colour Doppler US are very important in early and long-term allograft monitoring. This is because US provides a non-invasive, cheap, reproducible means to assess renal transplant (Tx) perfusion and drainage without nephrotoxicity and radiation which can be performed at the bedside or even intraoperatively if necessary (Figure 2.1). Doppler US is used to identify iliac and renal vessels. The resistive index (RI), a measure of blood flow, can be calculated as follows:

$$RI = (\text{peak systolic velocity} - \text{end diastolic velocity}) / \text{peak systolic velocity}$$

The normal value is ≈0.60, with 0.70 being around the upper limits of normal.

Normal peak systolic velocities for transplant renal arteries range up to 2.5 m/s [1]. Figure 2.2 shows normal renal vascular waveforms on Doppler US.

Vascular Complications

Transplant Renal Artery Stenosis

Transplant renal artery stenosis (TRAS) is a relatively common vascular complication

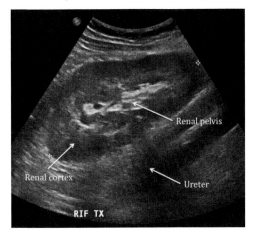

Figure 2.1 Normal greyscale ultrasound (US) of a renal allograft.

Radiology and Follow-up of Urologic Surgery, First Edition. Edited by Christopher Woodhouse and Alex Kirkham.
© 2018 John Wiley & Sons Ltd. Published 2018 by John Wiley & Sons Ltd.

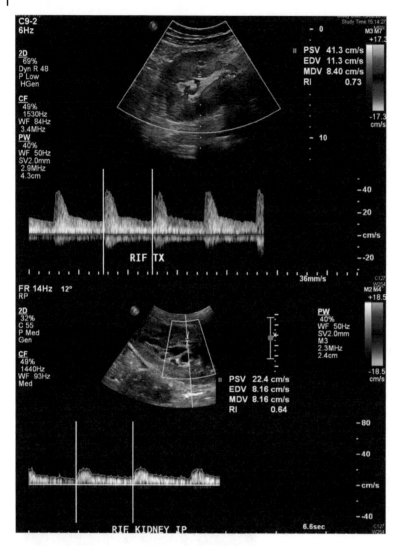

Figure 2.2 Doppler allograft US showing normal renal waveforms.

which can occur early or late [2]. Early recognition is important to prevent irreversible damage to the transplanted kidney and reduce patient morbidity [2, 3]. TRAS should be considered in patients with new onset and/or resistant hypertension, proteinuria and graft dysfunction. The cause of TRAS may be multifactorial including surgical technique, type of allograft, atherosclerosis and immunological factors as well as endothelial damage from calcineurin inhibitors [3, 4]. The most common situation is stenosis at the arterial anastomosis. This occurs more commonly with small arteries, especially if there

are multiple transplant renal arteries and if there is no aortic (Carrel) patch or if the aortic patch used had pre-existing atheromatous renal ostial stenosis. Occasionally, an existing arterial stenosis closer to the renal hilum becomes apparent post transplant. Rarely, a sharp kink in the Tx artery occurs as a result of incorrect positioning of the Tx kidney and/or Tx artery relative to the iliac artery [3].

Although Doppler US can be technically challenging, peak systolic velocity is the most sensitive criterion for the diagnosis of TRAS (Figure 2.3) [5].

Figure 2.3 Transplant renal artery stenosis (TRAS) Doppler waveform. US demonstrates severe elevation of systolic velocity at nearly 500 cm/s.

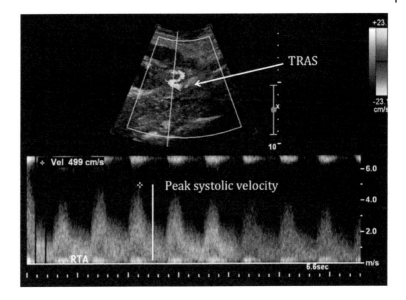

If Doppler US is abnormal, non-gadolinium magnetic resonance imaging (MRI) is performed to define the anatomy, confirm the diagnosis and guide subsequent management. Digital subtraction angiography is the 'gold standard' for the diagnosis of TRAS. It facilitates pressure measurements across a stenosis to confirm a diagnosis. It also permits interventional procedures such as percutaneous balloon angioplasty, with or without arterial stenting, to treat TRAS [1].

Surgical correction is reserved for patients unsuccessfully treated with interventional radiology methods (Figure 2.4).

Transplant Renal Vein Thrombosis

Transplant renal vein thrombosis (RVT) occurs in 0.3–3% of renal transplant patients [6]. Presentation is with acute pain and swelling over the graft as a result of abrupt non-function, typically on days 1–8 postoperatively. It can progress rapidly to rupture,

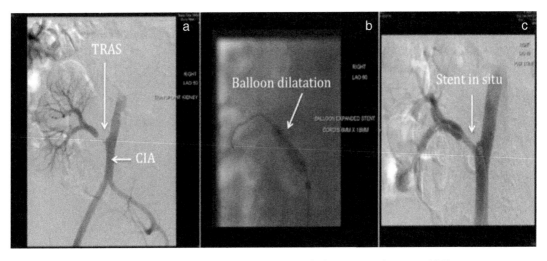

Figure 2.4 (a) Angiographic visualisation of TRAS at its junction with the common iliac artery (CIA). (b) Angioplasty and balloon dilatation of stenotic segment. (c) Transplant (Tx) renal artery stent insertion.

haemorrhage, and shock. Without a high index of suspicion, renal graft thrombosis can quickly lead to graft loss [1]. Reasons for RVT include poor anastomotic surgical technique, multiple transplant renal veins, kinking of the vessels during allograft positioning and ilio-femoral thrombosis. Predisposing risk factors include perioperative haemodynamic status (such as hypotension/hypoperfusion), prolonged ischaemia time, hypercoagulable recipient and acute rejection [7–10].

Renal duplex scanning is a useful non-invasive tool. Diagnosis is suggested by reversed arterial flow (Figure 2.5a), loss of venous flow on Doppler studies (Figure 2.5b) or evidence of a dilated renal vein with thrombosis within. If clinical suspicion of thrombosis is strong, angiographic contrast studies should be performed-immediately [6].

Transplant Renal Artery Thrombosis

Transplant renal artery thrombosis (RAT) occurs at sites of arterial damage. This may occur during harvest, benching or clamping of the vessels. Thrombosis is most commonly seen at areas of stenosis (Figure 2.6). Risk factors include multiple donor renal

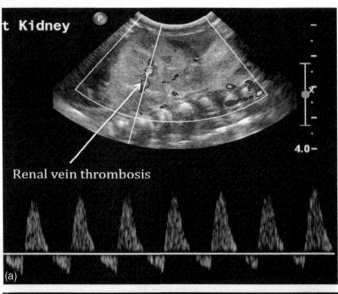

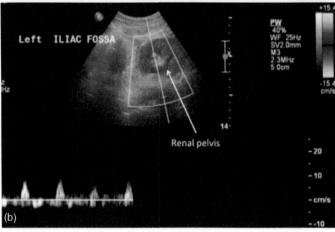

Figure 2.5 (a) Transplant renal vein thrombosis. Decreased venous blood flow to main renal vein at the hilum. Abnormal waveform showing reversed arterial flow. (b) Renal vein thrombosis and absent venous Doppler flow.

Figure 2.6 Transplant renal artery thrombosis (RAT) in a lower pole segmental artery.

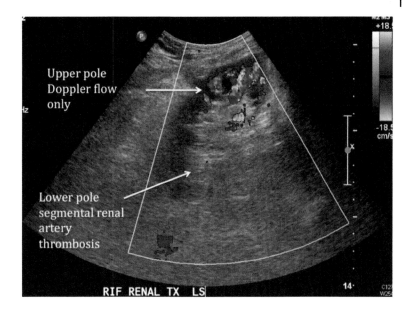

arteries, hypercoagubility, prolonged cold ischaemia time, delayed graft function and pre-transplant peritoneal dialysis [11].

Arteriovenous Fistula

Percutaneous renal biopsies provide key diagnostic information during investigation of transplant dysfunction. Iatrogenic renal vascular complications, however, do occur post renal biopsy, including pseudo-aneurysm, arteriovenous (AVF) and arteriocalyceal (ACF) fistulae (Figure 2.7) [12]. Their significance usually depends on their location and size and many are clinically unimportant [13]. Severe bleeding and persistent haematuria, widened pulse pressure, tachycardia and high-flow shunting require active management. Most commonly, treatment is with angiographic evaluation and endovascular embolisation. Rarely, partial or total nephrectomy or arterial ligation may be necessary [12, 13].

Follow-up

Close monitoring of parameters such as renal function and blood pressure are necessary following treatment of all vascular complications. Follow-up imaging is arranged on a

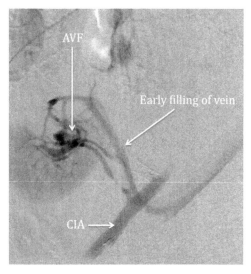

Figure 2.7 Iatrogenic arteriovenous fistula (AVF) from the CIA following transplant renal biopsy.

clinical and case-by-case basis. In general, an annual renal Doppler US is performed.

Urological Complications

Urological complications occur in 2.5–30% of renal transplant recipients [14]. Figures 2.8–2.14 in the following sections show how commonly occurring problems can be identified.

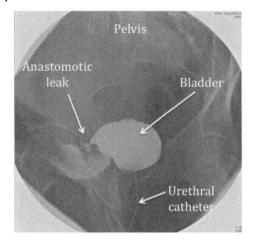

Figure 2.8 Cystogram image showing extravasation of urine at uretero-vesical anastomosis.

Ureteric Complications

Anastomotic Urinary Leak or Urinoma

The routine use of a Tx ureteric stent, tension-free well-vascularised mucosa to mucosa anastomosis, optimal organ positioning and bladder catheterisation all aim to protect the uretero-vesical anastomosis. Despite this, the literature reports urinary leak in 1.8–5.4% of cases (Figure 2.8). Other than surgical technique, the most common risk factors are donor age, multiple donor arteries, steroids and delayed graft function [15].

Once identified, management is dependent on the severity of the leak. Bladder catheterisation with maintenance of a ureteric stent and perinephric drain may allow a small

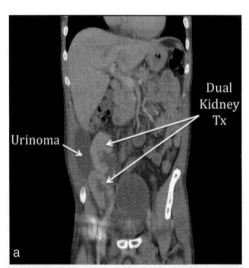

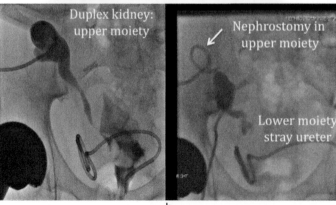

Figure 2.9 (a) CT scan showing urine leak of a missed duplex ureter from the lower of two dual kidney transplants. (b) Antegrade study showing the 'stray' duplex ureter not identified peroperatively.

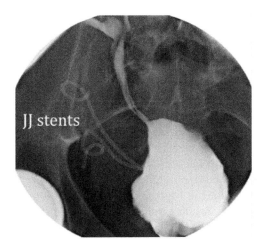

Figure 2.10 Dual kidney transplant with dual duplex ureters. The lower kidney duplex ureters have JJ stents in situ.

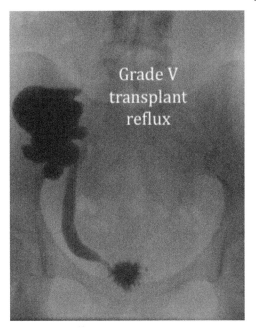

Figure 2.12 Micturating cysto-urethrogram (MCUG): right grade V transplant reflux.

defect to heal within 2–3 weeks. Interval cystogram can be performed to identify if there is ongoing extravasation of contrast. If no further leak is demonstrated, the catheter and stent can be removed. Ongoing clinical assessment and renal transplant US are used to identify signs of sepsis or ureteric obstruction. For larger anastomotic defects or persistent leaks, ureteric re-implantation is necessary. Follow-up with cystogram, retrograde studies or CT urogram can be used to confirm an intact anastomosis.

Missed Duplex Transplant Ureter

Ureteric duplication is the most commonly seen renal anomaly. It is found in 0.6–1.0% of donor kidneys [16]. The ureter may be partially or completely duplicated. Whilst duplex ureteric implantations potentially lend themselves to increased patient morbidity, case series in the literature show duplex kidneys to be safe for transplantation. Awareness of the possibility of a duplex ureter is important during donor kidney benching. This is to avoid complications from missed ureter and subsequent ureteric leak (Figure 2.9).

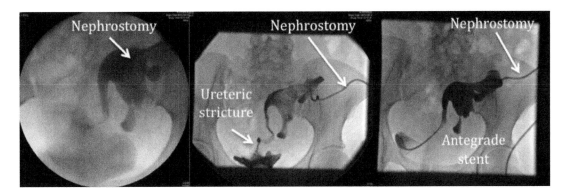

Figure 2.11 Serial nephrostogram images of ureteric obstruction secondary to ureteric stricture and subsequent antegrade stent insertion.

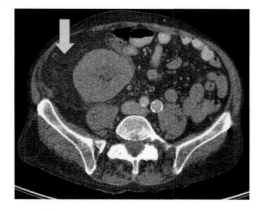

Figure 2.13 CT scan showing perinephric stranding indicating Tx pyelonephritis (arrow).

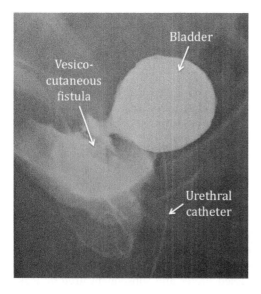

Figure 2.14 Cystogram showing a vesico-cutaneous fistula post renal transplant.

Extended donor criteria have led to an increase in the renal donor pool. This includes the use of dual kidney transplants in a single patient. The incidence of dual Tx kidneys both having duplex ureters is tiny. Figure 2.10 shows a patient successfully transplanted in this situation.

Ureteric Stenosis
Ureteric stenosis occurs in 2.4–6.5% of Tx cases [15]. Commonly, an ischaemic ureteric stricture ensues following tissue de-vascularisation or rejection although BK

viraemia is also a known precipitant [17]. Presentation is with renal graft dysfunction and decreased urine output. US shows graft hydronephrosis. Initially, a nephrostomy is inserted followed by an antegrade nephrostogram and often antegrade stent insertion (Figure 2.11). Whilst balloon dilatation may have a role, definitive management more often requires ureteric re-implantation. Success with balloon dilatation is variable and one should be mindful of the possibility of recurrent stricture formation or initial failure. Regular renal function tests and allograft US after balloon dilatation will confirm successful management or re-emergent hydronephrosis.

Transplant Ureteric Reflux
Despite improved intra- and extravesical uretero-vesicostomy techniques, a degree of reflux is common with transplant ureteric implantation. Despite this, no specific transplant reflux grading system exists. The international radiographic vesico-ureteric reflux grading system extrapolated from the non-transplant paediatric population is applied (Figure 2.12) [18].

The presence of reflux on its own does not mandate treatment. However, transplant pyelonephritis with accompanying renal dysfunction indicates high risk for renal graft loss and therefore intervention may be needed (Figure 2.13). In such cases a dimercaptosuccinic acid (DMSA) scan should be performed after the acute phase of infection has been treated. This defines areas of persistent scarring of the transplant cortex. Where possible, endo-urological submucosal injection at the transplant ureteric orifice is used as first line management for reflux. In severe or persistent cases, ureteric re-implantation is required.

Bladder Complications

Urinary Fistulae
Formation of a urinary fistula presents complex problems and high morbidity following transplant surgery. The most common sites

of uretero-cutaneous or vesico-cutaneous fistulae are at the uretero-vesicostomy or the ureter itself (Figure 2.14). Causative factors include poor surgical technique, ureteric ischaemia, acute rejection and neuropathic bladder [19]. Whilst small fistulas can be managed with temporary urine diversion techniques, definitive management of larger defects is with surgical excision of the fistula tract and repair. Postoperative outcome can be confirmed with endoscopic retrograde studies or a cystogram.

General Complications

Lymphocoeles

Many lymphocoeles are detected on US (Figure 2.15a) and may be asymptomatic. Symptomatic patients present most commonly with abdominal pain, lower limb oedema, graft dysfunction or deep vein thrombosis. Lymphocoeles arise through leakage from lymphatic vessels of the transplanted kidney or those surrounding the iliac vessels of the recipient [20].

Renal Transplant Stone Disease

Urolithiasis in the renal Tx patient is either de novo allograft stone formation (with no prior evidence of donor urolithiasis) or stones that are 'donor gifted' (i.e. transferred with the transplant kidney).

The incidence of new onset stone disease in renal transplant patients is low, ranging between 0.4% and 6% [21]. Because of allograft denervation, one must be aware that patients may not present with typical symptoms of renal colic and are therefore at risk of ureteric obstruction. The exact mechanism

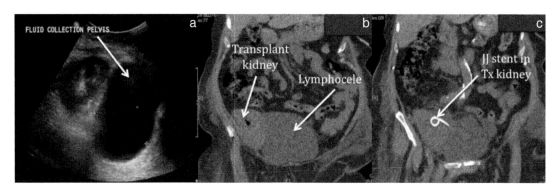

Figure 2.15 (a) US showing lymphocoele. (b, c) CT confirmation of a perinephric, extravesical collection in which the ureteric stent is not seen to be present.

Figure 2.16 Arrows highlighting stones present in right iliac fossa (RIF) transplant kidney prior to treatment. X-ray of the kidneys, ureter and bladder (KUB) shows how stones are often difficult to ascertain on a plain film (a) because of the overlying bone. They are clearly seen on CT (b).

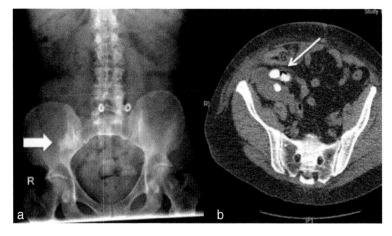

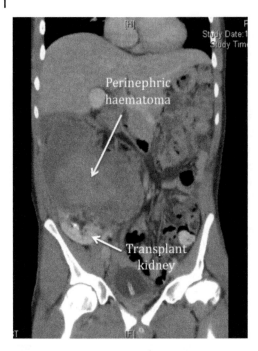

Figure 2.17 CT scan showing large haematoma secondary to graft rupture following blunt trauma to the abdomen. Areas of high and low density are seen within the collection. The high density is a typical feature of a bleed.

of allograft stone formation is not known [20]. However, calcineurin inhibitor (CNI) usage is known to affect metabolic homeostasis causing hypocitraturia, hyperkalaemia, hyperoxaluria, hypercalciuria and hypomagnesaemia. These imbalances predispose to stone formation [21]. Other factors such as vesico-ureteric reflux, urinary tract infections, renal tubular acidosis and low urinary pH also have a role. Correction of causative factors and metabolic imbalances forms an essential part of management. Stones are treated by endo-urological, percutaneous, lithotripsy or open surgery, depending on size, location and ease of access through the transplant ureter (Figure 2.16) [22].

Better screening of deceased and living donor organs has led to improved pre-operative detection of 'donor gifted' stones and ex vivo ureteroscopy can render a kidney stone-free prior to transplantation [23].

Renal Transplant Trauma

Because of allograft positioning, the kidney is particularly vulnerable to blunt, as well as penetrating, trauma (Figures 2.17 and 2.18). A high index of suspicion is required as acute rejection, graft rupture and graft loss can occur.

Oncological Complications

Transplant Renal Cell Carcinoma

Renal cell carcinoma (RCC) is more common in the native kidneys than the allograft

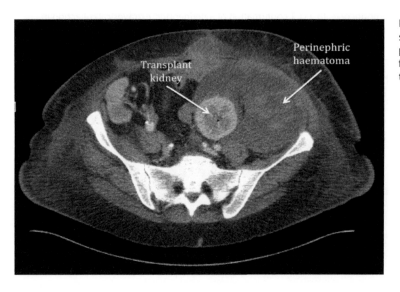

Figure 2.18 CT scan showing large perinephric haematoma following a renal transplant biopsy.

Figure 2.19 Contrast-enhanced CT scan showing subtle difference in enhancement of the small renal mass. This is likely to be a renal cell carcinoma (RCC).

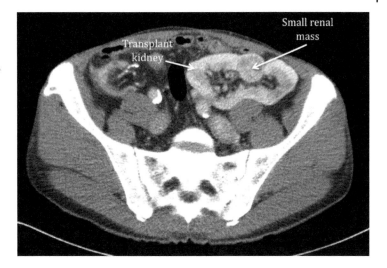

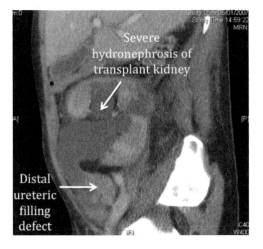

Figure 2.20 Contrast-enhanced CT scan showing a filling defect in the distal Tx ureter causing Tx hydronephrosis. *Source:* Olsburgh *et al.* [26]. Reproduced with permission of John Wiley and Sons.

itself [24]. The incidence of de novo RCC is low at 0.19–0.5% [25]. Investigation is best carried out with contrast-enhanced CT scan, if the patient's renal function allows it (Figure 2.19). US, non-contrast CT or MRI may be used if graft function is poor.

Whilst renal transplant nephrectomy remains the treatment of choice in these cases, newer surgical techniques and close follow-up have paved the way to possible partial nephrectomies even in the renal transplant population (see Chapter 1).

Transplant Ureteric Transitional Cell Carcinoma

Transitional cell carcinoma (TCC) of the transplant ureter (TCCtu) is rare. Presentation in most cases is with graft dysfunction and haematuria. This should always be investigated urgently. An US followed by a subsequent contrast-enhanced CT urogram is the gold standard. Transplant hydronephrosis is often seen secondary to TCCtu obstruction (Figure 2.20). This requires either a percutaneous nephrostomy or JJ stent insertion in the first instance whilst an appropriate oncological management plan is being considered.

Early detection of TCCtu enables potentially curative ureteric resection, preservation of a functioning Tx and urinary tract reconstruction [25]. In some cases, however, a transplant nephrectomy and return to dialysis are unavoidable.

Conclusions

The breath of potential complications following renal transplantation is vast. We describe a select few of the commonly arising problems. Clearly, appropriate radiological investigation has a pivotal role in the early detection and management of these complications.

References

1 Baxter GM. Ultrasound of renal transplantation. *Clin Radiol.* 2001; 56(10): 802–818.

2 Fervenza F, Lafayette R, Alfrey E, Petersen J. Renal artery stenosis in kidney transplants. *Am J Kidney Dis.* 1998; 31(1): 142–148.

3 Wong W, Fynn SP, Higgins RM, *et al.* Transplant renal artery stenosis in 77 patients: does it have an immunological cause? *Transplantation.* 1996; (61): 215–219.

4 Patel U, Khaw K, Hughes N. Doppler ultrasound for detection of renal transplant artery stenosis: threshold peak systolic velocity needs to be higher in a low-risk or surveillance population. *Clin Radiol.* 2003; 58(10): 772–777.

5 Rerolle JP, Antoine C, Raynaud A, *et al.* Successful endoluminal thrombo-aspiration of renal graft venous thrombosis. *Transpl Int.* 2000; 13(1): 82–86.

6 Merion RM, Calne RY. Allograft renal vein thrombosis. *Transpl Proc.* 1985; 17: 1746–1750.

7 Hilfiker ML, Feddersen RM, Gibe LJ, Smith AY, Harford AM, Sterling WA. Allograft renal vein thrombosis in a kidney with two veins. *Transplantation.* 1992; 54: 738–739.

8 Bakir N, Sluiter WJ, Ploeg RJ, van son WJ, Tegzess AM. Primary renal graft thrombosis. *Nephrol Dial Transpl.* 1986; 11: 140–147.

9 Penny MJ, Nankivell BJ, Disney AP, Byth K, Chapman JR. Renal graft thrombosis: a survey of 134 consecutive cases. *Transplantation.* 1994; 58: 565–569.

10 Gruber SA, Pescovitz MD, Simmons RL, *et al.* Thromboembolic complications in renal allograft recipients: a report from the prospective randomized study of cyclosporine versus azathioprine-antilymphocyte globulin. *Transplantation.* 1987; 44: 775–778.

11 Fallahzadeh MK, Yatavelli RK, Kumar A, *et al.* Acute transplant renal artery thrombosis due to distal renal artery stenosis: a case report and review of the literature. *J Nephropathol.* 2014; 3(3): 105–108.

12 Loffroy R, Guiu B, Lambert A, *et al.* Management of post-biopsy renal allograft arteriovenous fistulas with selective arterial embolization: immediate and long-term outcomes. *Clin Radiol.* 2008; 63(6): 657–665.

13 Paschalis-Purtak K, Januszewicz, Rokicki A, *et al.* Arteriovenous fistula of the kidney: a case report of 47-year-old female patient treated by embolisation. *J Hum Hypertens.* 2003; 17: 293–296.

14 Slagt I, Ijzermans, Visser L, *et al.* Independent risk factors for urological complications after deceased donor kidney transplantation. *PLoS ONE.* 2014; 9(3): e91211.

15 Berli JU, Montgomery JR, Segev DL, *et al.* Surgical management of early and late ureteral complications after renal transplantation: techniques and outcomes. *Clin Transplant.* 2015; 29: 26–33.

16 Alberts VP, Minnee RC, van Donselaare-van der Pant KA, *et al.* Duplicated ureters and renal transplantation: a case–control study and review of the literature. *Transplant Proc.* 2013; 45: 3239–3244.

17 Deepak KR, Gomez A, Tsang W, Shanberg A. Ureteric and urethral stenosis: a complication of BK virus infection in a paediatric renal transplant patient. *Pediatr Transplant.* 2007; 11(4): 433–435.

18 Lebowitz RL, Olbing H, Parkkulainen KV, Smellie JM, Tamminen-Möbius TE. International system of radiographic grading of vesicoureteric reflux. International Reflux Study in Children. *Paediatr Radiol.* 1985; 15(2): 105–109.

19 Basić D, Djokić JH, Milutinović D, Dzamic Z, Topuzović C, Pejcić T. Ureteral

fistulae after kidney transplantation: experience with 224 cases. *Acta Chir Iugosl.* 2011; 58(1): 89–94.

20 Sim A, Ng LG, Cheng C. Occurrence of a lymphocele following renal transplantation. *Singapore Med J.* 2013; 54(5): 259–262.

21 Savasci S, Bostanci Y, Ozden E, *et al.* Metabolic evaluation of kidney transplant recipients for stone disease and comparison with healthy controls and stone formers. *J Urol Surg.* 2015; 1: 28–32.

22 Breda A, Olsburgh J, Budde K, *et al.* European Association of Urology Guidelines: Renal transplantation, https://uroweb.org/guideline/renal-transplantation (accessed 2 June 2017).

23 Wong K, Olsburgh J. Management of stones in renal transplant. *Curr Opin Urol.* 2013; 23(2): 175–179.

24 Chapman JR, Webster AC, Wong G. Cancer in the transplant recipient. *Perspect Med.* 2013; 3(7).

25 Tillou X, Doerfler A, Collon S, *et al.* De novo kidney graft tumors: results from a multicentric retrospective national study. *Am J Transplant.* 2012; 12(12): 3308–3315.

26 Olsburgh J, Zakri RH, Horsfield C, *et al.* TCC in transplant ureter: when and when not to preserve the transplant kidney. *Am J Transplant.* 2016; 16(2): 704–711.

3

Imaging After Endo-urological Stone Treatment

Daron Smith and Clare Allen

Introduction

The surgical management of urinary tract stones has been revolutionised during the working lifetime of many senior urologists. Until about 1990, the huge majority of upper tract stones were removed by open surgery. Except with complex staghorn stones, it was usual for the patient to be rendered 'stone free' by a single procedure, albeit through an incision that was very much larger than the stones themselves. Nowadays, surgeons have a variety of minimally invasive procedures from which to choose, although some are less 'minimally invasive' than others. The most common unsatisfactory outcome is that the stone burden is not entirely removed; incomplete clearance has therefore become routine, providing the failure rate is within parameters acceptable to surgeons. The patient may regard failure to clear the stones as a complication, though may accept it providing the possibility was clearly explained in advance or the procedure was regarded as a part of a course of treatment.

The surgeon is therefore trying to select one of many possible techniques according to the nature of the stone burden, its position and the anatomy of the urinary tract. Unlike most of the other chapters in this book, the arrangement of sections in this one is to show the outcomes by these criteria and the techniques used, in addition to the more conventionally reported complications for other urological procedures such as death, structural damage and infection. Accordingly, it covers the endoscopic, fluoroscopic and postoperative appearances of the urinary tract as a consequence of stone disease, both following active treatment and from the potential consequences of conservative management during which secondary complications may occur. Specifically, the features following minimally invasive treatment with extracorporeal shock wave lithotripsy (ESWL), and of the surgical treatment by 'endoluminal endourology'– ureteroscopy (URS), flexible ureterorenoscopy (FURS; also known as retrograde intrarenal surgery, RIRS) and percutaneous nephrolithotomy (PCNL) – are discussed.

The Procedures

Conservative Management

Guidance for the decision to treat incidentally detected stones actively or to adopt an observational approach and treat if needs be can be derived from studies that detail the natural history of conservatively managed stones, in which 'progression' (i.e. stone growth, obstruction or pain) would lead to a change of tack from observation to intervention (Figure 3.1).

For patients presenting with asymptomatic renal stones, Kaplan–Meier analysis suggests that by 7.25 years of follow-up about 50% of all patients will have required no surgical

Radiology and Follow-up of Urologic Surgery, First Edition. Edited by Christopher Woodhouse and Alex Kirkham.
© 2018 John Wiley & Sons Ltd. Published 2018 by John Wiley & Sons Ltd.

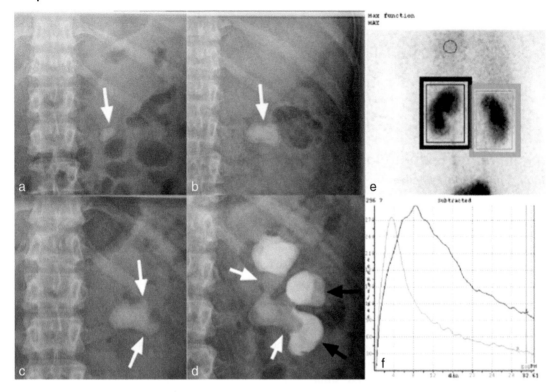

Figure 3.1 Conservative management of renal stone. These plain film images show a left renal pelvic stone (a, white arrow) gradually enlarging (b), then branching towards the inter- and lower-pole calyces (c, arrows). (d) An intravenous urogram (IVU) performed 18 months after the initial image, the relation of stone (white arrows) to calices (black arrows) is shown. (e,f) A MAG3 renogram at the time of the IVU shows that, despite the enlargement of the stone, at this stage there has been good preservation of function and that the left kidney (represented by the black line on the renogram curves) is unobstructed.

intervention and suffered no renal damage. Those with stones of >4 mm, in the lower pole or pelvis and associated with higher urinary calcium or uric acid were more likely to require surgical treatment [1].

In some patients therefore, observation by annual ultrasound (US) for 7 years could be offered and surgical intervention used for *significant* pain or stone growth. If the stone is not seen on ultrasound, a CT scan of the kidneys, ureters and bladder (KUB) may be needed, either to confirm its absence or to plan intervention if the patient remains symptomatic or has risk factors and therefore might opt for preventative intervention.

However, if preventative intervention is considered, it is important to balance the decision to treat against the knowledge that

intervention for asymptomatic renal stones carries risks, dependent on the magnitude of the treatment required. In a prospectively randomised trial comparing PCNL against ESWL with observation, PCNL had a 100% stone-free rate, with a 3% chance of a renal scar on follow-up dimercaptosuccinic acid (DMSA) scan, compared with a 3% chance of being stone free (due to spontaneous passage) at 1 year if observed, but with no scars. The worst outcome was in patients undergoing ESWL who had a 61.3% stone-free rate at 1 year, with four of 31 having additional treatment by PCNL or URS/FURS, and a scar by DMSA in 16% [2].

Conservative management is frequently used in the management of ureteric stones, where there is an adequate likelihood of

Figure 3.2 Ureteric colic, with spontaneous passage of stone. Unenhanced low dose CT shows a hydronephrotic left kidney (a, arrow) with a 3-mm stone (b, arrow, and in a coronal reconstruction, c) at the left vesico-ureteric junction (VUJ). The follow-up ultrasound (US) (d) shows an undilated kidney, with prominent ureteric jets at both the right (e) and left (f) ureteric orifices (red flares). These findings are consistent with the expected spontaneous passage of a small distal ureteric stone.

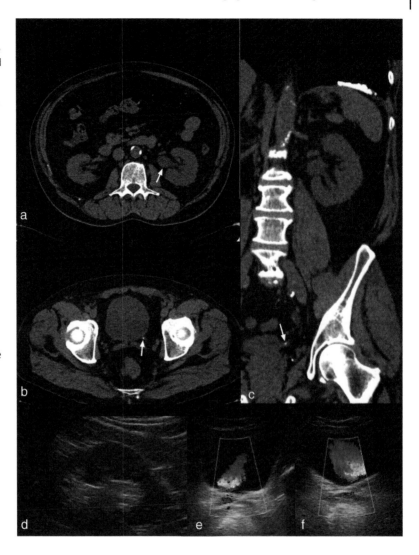

spontaneous stone passage (Figure 3.2). As with renal calculi, the size and position of the stone are key factors in the decision making: the smaller the stone and the lower in the ureter, the more likely it is to pass (Table 3.1) [3, 4]. After controlling the severe pain of ureteric colic at presentation, subsequent episodes of pain are not usually so intense (particularly as the patient now knows the cause) such that observation is still a reasonable option even in patients with a dramatic initial presentation.

Conservative management cannot be continued indefinitely, however, because of the risk of functional loss. Here stone size is not relevant but the period of obstruction is; patients whose stones pass within 14 days have 100% renal recovery, compared to only 65% of those that remain for more than 28 days. Upstream infection accelerates damage, and therefore needs immediate intervention, not only to preserve function but to prevent the serious complications of systemic inflammatory response syndrome (SIRS) and/or sepsis (Figure 3.3) [5]. For conservative management to be justified, monitoring must be sufficiently frequent to prevent a relatively simple stone becoming a kidney or even life-threatening problem.

Table 3.1 Likelihood of spontaneous passage of a ureteric stone by size and position on presentation.

Stone size (mm)	Spontaneous passage rate (%)	Stone position	Spontaneous passage rate (%)
1	87	Proximal ureter	48
2–4	76	Mid ureter	60
5–7	60	Distal ureter	75
7–9	48	VUJ	79
>9	25		

VUJ, vesicoureteric junction.
Source: Data from Coll *et al.* [4].

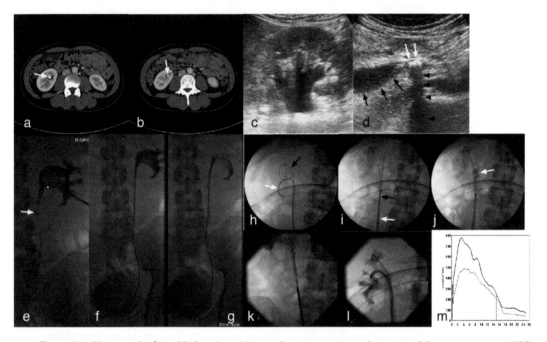

Figure 3.3 Obstructed infected kidney (requiring nephrostomy, antegrade stent and then ureteroscopy, URS). (a,b) The first two axial CT images show stones in multiple calyces (white arrows) of the right kidney. The patient subsequently presented with right loin pain, renal angle tenderness and a fever; US showed a dilated renal pelvis (c), with a dilated proximal ureter (d, black arrows), due to a stone in the proximal ureter (d, white arrows), including a prominent post-acoustic shadow (d, black arrowheads). This required the emergency insertion of a nephrostomy tube. When recovered, a nephrostogram was performed which shows drainage of contrast (e, black arrows) beyond the stone (e, white arrow) allowing an antegrade JJ stent to be placed (f) and the nephrostomy tube removed (g).
The patient was treated by flexible ureterorenoscopy (FURS) showing an initial safety wire (h, black arrow) alongside the stent (h, white arrow) and an access sheath (i, white arrow) inserted over a separate working guide wire over which the flexible ureterorenoscope was advanced (i, black arrow). Contrast via the scope showed some extravasation (j, arrow) consistent with ureteric trauma, requiring a further JJ stent for drainage at the end of the procedure. A 'second look' ureterorenoscopy was performed, showing the ureter retained a normal calibre (k) allowing access of the ureterorenoscope to the kidney (l) and with subsequent unobstructed drainage by MAG3 renography (m) in which the right kidney is represented by the dotted line (i.e. that there is no ureteric stricture).

An US for patients with a dilated upper tract should ideally be performed no later than 2 weeks after presentation and stone removal arranged if the dilatation has not resolved. If there is any doubt about the presence of obstruction, a MAG3 scan should be performed. Up to 28% of patients intended to be followed with conservative intent have been shown to have 'silent' loss of function at presentation (Figure 3.4). Stone removal within 7 days gives better functional recovery than if it is delayed [6].

Ureteric Stones: Results and Complications

Extracorporeal shock wave lithotripsy

If ESWL (Figure 3.5) is to be undertaken for ureteric stones, early treatment has an advantage for stone clearance over delayed intervention. In a prospective study of 94 patients with at least one episode of colic secondary to a solitary unilateral proximal ureteric stone (mean stone size 7.9 ± 2.3 mm), patients treated within 24 hours had a mean time to stone clearance of 6.4 ± 6.3 days, compared with 16.0 ± 7.8 days if treated beyond the first day [7].

This may be a result of gradual impaction of the stone with time. This theory is supported by the finding that ureteric wall thickness at the impaction site is the key variable that predicts ESWL success [8]. In addition, patients with a solitary lumbar ureteric stone without hydronephrosis have higher stone-free rates after ESWL than those with dilatation (89.1% stone free vs 80.3% stone free). Patients with hydronephrosis (i.e. those more likely to have a long-standing and/or impacted stone) had a greater need for repeat treatment (2.4 vs 1.7 sessions) and a longer time before stone clearance is achieved (16.2 vs 11.6 days) [9].

In turn, this is consistent with long-standing data regarding repeat treatment with ESWL, whereby a 68% stone-free rate after initial treatment increased to 76% if a second treatment is performed, but only to 77% overall if a third treatment is given [10].

This situation is not improved by the placement of a JJ stent – a systematic review of eight randomised controlled trials (RCTs; 876 patients, 453 stented and 423 unstented) showed no difference in stone-free rate between stented and unstented patients (relative rate, RR 0.97) at a cost of a significantly higher risk of lower urinary tract symptoms in the stented group (RR 4.10) [11].

These data demonstrate that, if ESWL is going to be effective, it is best done early. If clearance is not achieved in one or two sessions, neither positioning of a JJ stent nor more ESWL is likely to yield further benefit.

Ureteroscopy

Ureteroscopy has been shown to be an effective and safe intervention for ureteric stones in two recent studies involving more than 17 000 patients. Using data from the Clinical Research Office of the Endourology Society (CROES) ureteroscopy database, stone clearance can be expected in approximately 95% of distal ureteric stones, 90% of mid ureteric stones and in 85% of proximal ureteric stones [12].

Complication rates are now acceptably low, with minor intraoperative issues such as mucosal abrasions or bleeding accounting for over two-thirds. More serious events such as ureteric perforation (0.7%), extra-ureteric stone migration (0.1%) and ureteric avulsion are reassuringly rare (0.04%) (Figure 3.6) [13]. Accordingly, ureteroscopic management is an increasingly popular intervention, with nearly a 50% increase between 2009–2010 and 2014–2015 [14].

Stone size and location, impaction, operation time and surgeon experience are factors influencing the rate of complications [13]. A 'favourable' ureteroscopy is a single procedure that achieves a stone-free patient with no complications. In a series of 841 patients undergoing 908 ureteroscopic procedures, this was achieved in 83%. Complications occurred in 6.7% overall. Risk factors for an unfavourable result were proximal ureteric stones (RR 4), an inexperienced surgeon

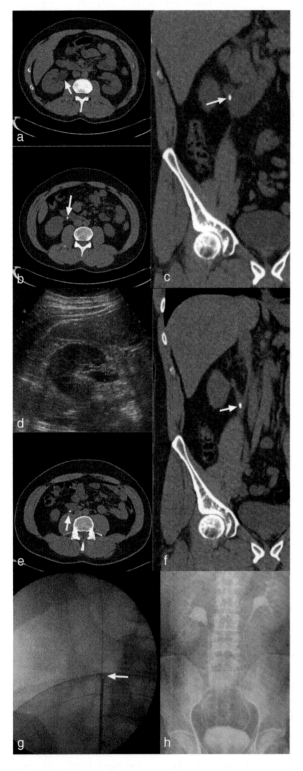

Figure 3.4 Ureteric colic, with failure of stone to pass. Unenhanced low dose CT shows a hydronephrotic right kidney in axial section (a) with a 5-mm stone (arrow) in the right proximal ureter in axial (b) and coronal sections (c). Although the patient was pain free, the follow-up US (d) shows a mildly dilated kidney in axial view (marker crosses) for which a repeat CT (e,f) shows the stone remains. This patient required ureteroscopy and laser stone fragmentation (g) to clear the stone (just visible at the tip of the ureteroscope, white arrow). (h) An IVU was performed for follow-up (this is not a commonly used test nowadays) but clearly demonstrates normal symmetrical excretion of contrast, and bilateral undilated/unobstructed ureteric drainage. These images demonstrate the potential risk of 'silent obstruction' in a patient who is asymptomatic, but who does not experience the passage of the stone, and the importance of follow-up imaging to ensure a stone-free state.

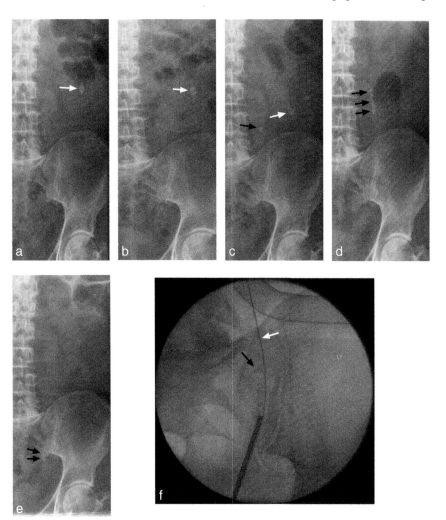

Figure 3.5 Ureteric steinstrasse requiring URS and laser to clear. These images show the progressive fragmentation of a left lower pole stone (a, white arrow) by extracorporeal shock wave lithotripsy (ESWL), demonstrating fragments initially in the lower pole (b, white arrow) which are further fragmented after additional ESWL (c, white arrow) on follow-up imaging with a 'lead fragment' in the ureter (c, black arrow). The stone fragments then accumulate behind this leading fragment to create a ureteric steinstrasse (d, black arrows). Although this showed some progression towards the middle/lower third of the ureter (e, black arrow), a ureteroscopy was performed to clear the stones. In this image, a safety guidewire (f, white arrow) and a 'stone cone®' (Boston Scientific) can be seen (f, black arrow) above the tip of the ureteroscope.

(RR 2.5), an impacted stone (RR 1.8) and stone width (RR 1.2) [15].

In another series, ureteroscopic success was negatively associated with primary stone size, total stone number and cumulative stone burden. Insertion of a JJ stent increased stone clearance to 97% of patients compared with 87% without a prior stent [16].

Antegrade ureteroscopy via the kidney can be considered. Operating time is longer but stone-free rates are significantly better for stones >15 mm above the level of L4, when compared with retrograde URS. This may be caused by retropulsion of stones, because the clearance rates were similar for stones below L4, with retropulsion seen in less than

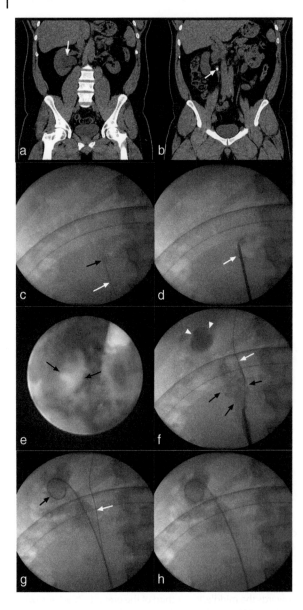

Figure 3.6 Impacted proximal ureteric stone. These images show the challenge of the impacted large proximal ureteric stone, demonstrated by a hydronephrotic right kidney on CT in coronal section (a) with a large stone (arrow) in the right proximal ureter (b). It was not possible to pass a safety wire (c, arrow) beyond the stone (c, black arrow), so a ureteroscope was passed alongside the wire (seen buckling into an 'S' shape; d, arrow). A hydrophilic-tipped wire was aimed to pass the stone (almost 'epithelialised' from being long-standing and impacted; ureteroscope image in e). A contrast study via the ureteroscope shows this wire had perforated the ureter (f, white arrow), with extravasation (f, black arrows), although some contrast was evident in a dilated calyx (f, white arrowheads). Leaving the perforating wire in situ, the ureteroscope was repassed, and the stone fragmented with a laser, allowing a second wire to be inserted to the renal pelvis. The perforating wire (g, white arrow) was left in situ ('plugging the hole') until a JJ stent was inserted over the second wire (g, black arrow), at which point the perforating wire was safely removed (h).

10%, compared with just under 50% for those higher than the upper border of the fourth lumbar vertebra [17].

Renal Stones: Results and Complications

Flexible Ureterorenoscopy

UK national statistics have shown that, whilst the rate of ESWL for stones remained stable, and the number of open surgical procedures continued to decline to just 30 cases in 2014–2015, the number of FURS treatments doubled in the UK from 3267 to 6631 between 2009 and 2015 [14].

CROES data from 1210 patients undergoing FURS for solitary kidney stone across 114 worldwide centres showed that operation time positively correlated with stone size, and the stone-free rate negatively correlated with stone size, such that 90% of stones <10 mm in size were cleared in a single session, reducing to 80% for stones <15 mm, and down to 30% clearance at the initial operation in stones >20 mm in size. Although no difference in overall complication rates was noted, stones >20 mm had a higher probability of fever [18]. For the larger stones (mean size 30 mm), a 91% clearance rate has been reported but at the expense of long operative times (up to 138 minutes) and a median of two procedures per patient [19].

In such cases, access sheaths are generally useful, to aid vision through better irrigation

whilst helping to maintain a low intrarenal pressure, and to allow multiple trips of the scope to and from the kidney if stone fragments are being retrieved. However, this comes at the potential cost of ureteric wall injury, which has been reported to be more prevalent than previously considered, occurring to some extent in 46.5%, and classed as severe (involving smooth muscle) in 13.3% (Figure 3.7). Risk factors include being male, older and not having a prior JJ stent [20].

FURS is particularly useful in complex situations for which ESWL might take multiple

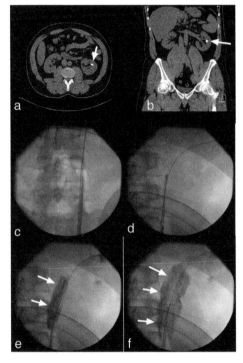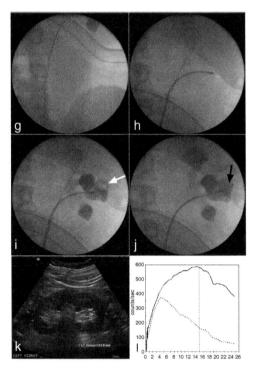

Figure 3.7 Ureteric trauma from an access sheath. These images show the potential for ureteric injury to be caused by larger calibre instruments, in this case a ureteric access sheath. The stones were in a calyceal diverticulum, shown in axial (a) and coronal (b) CT images, such that a ureteric access sheath was inserted (c) to facilitate irrigation and drainage, thereby improving the endoscopic view. The ureter was tight, precluding advancement of the ureterorenoscope to the kidney. (d) Contrast injected via the scope (intended to show the path of the ureter to the renal pelvis) demonstrated extravasation medially (e, white arrows) and then expanding across or down the retroperitoneum (f, white arrows). A JJ stent was placed, and easier access achieved subsequently – the access sheath is shown in (g), allowing the ureterorenoscope to reach the interpole of the left kidney (h). The stones are visible as a filling-defect (i, white arrow) which is no longer seen after the diverticulum has been identified with a guide wire (j, black arrow) and the ureterorenoscope then passed into this after widening the neck of the diverticulum with a laser, and fragmenting or retrieving the stones. Follow-up US shows good renal parenchyma no hydronephrosis or stone recurrence (k). The MAG3 renogram showed normal split function with a 'dilated-unobstructed' appearance to the drainage curves (the left kidney is represented by the black line in l).

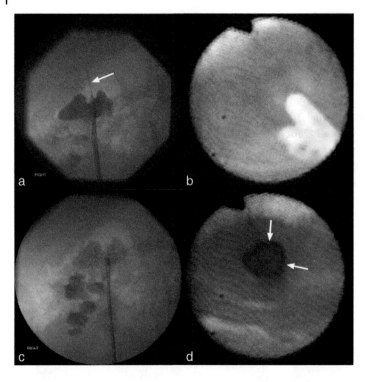

Figure 3.8 Upper calyceal wire perforation. These images show an upper pole wire perforation (a, arrow) evident beyond the contrast in the upper calyces on fluoroscopy (a) and endoscopic view (b). When the wire was withdrawn under vision, a small blood clot formed at the site of the perforation (d, arrows), such that there was no contrast extravasation into the renal parenchyma or around the renal capsule (c).

sessions and/or not achieve stone clearance and PCNL would require two or more punctures.

For stones in multiple locations within the kidney, particularly in larger volume burdens, a stone-free rate of 64.7% after one procedure rising to 92.2% after two procedures can be achieved. Patients with a total stone burden <20 mm were 100% stone free, compared to 85.1% in patients with >20 mm [21].

Similarly, patients with bilateral stones can be treated simultaneously with FURS, starting with the symptomatic side, or the side with the greater stone burden if asymptomatic. In findings similar to the data above, the stone-free rate was 100% for a stone burden <25 mm and 80% for a stone burden ≥25 mm. If a bilateral procedure is performed, then at least one JJ stent will be needed to avoid the potential for postoperative anuric renal failure requiring emergency stent insertion subsequently [22]. Stents are also required for any unexpected intraoperative issue, including the risk of postoperative infection, to maintain ureteric drainage

and thereby provide a more predictable postoperative course (Figures 3.8 and 3.9).

Unlike ESWL, in which stone-free rates are cumulatively adversely affected if the infundibulo-pelvic angle is less than 90 degrees, or its length and width >3 cm or <5 mm, respectively, successful stone clearance by FURS is possible even if two of these factors are unfavourable (although it may be sensible to relocate the stones into a more suitable location within the kidney for laser treatment and/or stone fragment extraction). If all three factors are unfavourable, a percutaneous approach may be preferable [23].

Percutaneous Surgery

The finding that stone clearance rates decrease for both ESWL and FURS for stones >15 mm has been confirmed by a systematic review comparing ESWL, FURS and PCNL for the treatment of ≤20 mm lower pole stones in adults (7 RCTs involving 691 patients) comparing stone-free rate at 3 months or less. It confirmed a higher chance of clearance by PCNL (risk ratio 2.04; 95%

Figure 3.9 These images show the potential for more adverse consequences from a parenchymal wire perforation than demonstrated in Figure 3.8. In this case, the safety wire and working wires are seen in the upper calyx (a), following which an access sheath (b, white arrow) has been advanced over the hydrophilic-tipped wire (b, black arrow), which can be seen to coil safely back towards the renal pelvis. The other wire (a standard PTFE wire) has continued beyond its original position as the sheath was advanced (b, arrowhead). This wire shows a kink (c, arrowhead) and can be seen to extend beyond the collecting system when contrast is instilled via the ureterorenoscope (d, arrowhead). This is confirmed by direct visualisation with the ureterorenoscope in the relevant calyx (e), leaving the perforating wire in situ whilst the procedure is completed (f). In this case, when the perforating wire was withdrawn, the collecting system rapidly filled with blood (g, arrowheads) and demonstrated a subcapsular collection of contrast on the final image with a JJ stent in situ (h, arrowheads). A second 're-look' procedure subsequently showed a normal collecting system, with no residual blood clot and no ongoing contrast leak.

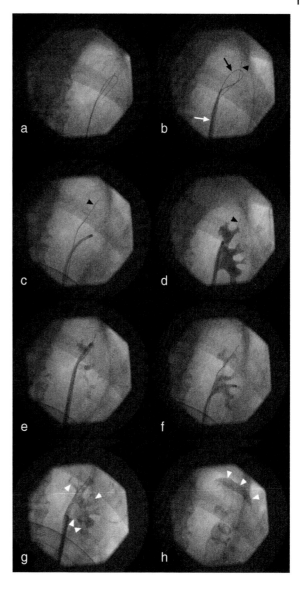

CI 1.50–2.77) over ESWL and FURS (risk ratio 1.31; 95% CI 1.08–1.59) over ESWL. However, the benefit was 'markedly less for ≤10 mm stones', suggesting that ESWL should still be the first line treatment for smaller renal stones [24].

Similar findings were published in two additional meta-analyses by Lee *et al.* [25] and Srisubat *et al.* [26]. In the former, PCNL and ureterorenoscopy were more effective than ESWL therapy alone for lower pole stones (risk ratio of being stone free for PCNL was 2.19 and for FURS was 1.23). However, ESWL can be made more effective with adjunctive manoeuvres such as diuresis and inversion, improving its risk ratio to 1.30 over ESWL alone [25]. In the latter study, a Cochrane review of ESWL vs PCNL vs FURS for kidney stones (five RCTs comprising 338 patients, four studies compared ESWL with PCNL and one compared ESWL with FURS), ESWL was shown to be less effective than PCNL but not significantly different from FURS, but with a shorter hospital stay and duration of treatment with ESWL. However, ESWL is nine times more likely to require additional ('auxiliary') procedures than FURS or PCNL [26].

Data from the CROES Global PCNL Study showed that ultrasound-guided access reduces puncture time and radiation exposure. The likelihood of postoperative fever was 10.5% (antibiotic prophylaxis gives a threefold lower postoperative fever rate) and the overall risk of bleeding was directly related to the size of the dilatation with larger calibre access having a higher chance of bleeding, hence the current trend towards smaller tracks for PCNL (Figure 3.10). However, even small tracks can damage adjacent structures with a small incidence of puncturing the thorax (Figure 3.11). This study demonstrated that complications were more likely in patients with severe chronic kidney disease, those with a solitary kidney (who have a tendency to a reduced stone-free rate and more bleeding) and in elderly patients. Obese patients have a similar outcome to the general population, although the 'super-obese (BMI >40)' have a higher chance of more severe complications [27].

Staghorn stones represent a particular challenge, both for intervention and conservative management. The latter has been known for at least 50 years to carry a high risk of death or renal failure and should only be considered in patients with extensive co-morbidity, otherwise stone treatment should be attempted. Whilst surgery on staghorn calculi is often difficult and complete eradication of the stone can be impossible, even if only the renal pelvis is cleared, the renal-related mortality is reduced to only 3% [28, 29].

Following PCNL, the question of tube drainage of the kidney remains an important decision. A nephrostomy is indicated for significant blood loss, urine extravasation, ureteric obstruction and risk of sepsis secondary to infected stones and is sensible following surgery on a solitary kidney. It is also valuable in patients who may have residual stones, and who might benefit

from a 'second look' procedure using the nephrostomy tract to regain renal access for the additional stone(s) to be removed. In patients with normal renal function, a single tract procedure, complete stone clearance and minimal bleeding, omitting a nephrostomy gives less postoperative pain and a shorter hospital stay [30].

Complications and Follow-up

It will be seen from the above data that complications, including failure to achieve stone clearance, can be minimised by good training and proper selection of procedures: matching the surgeon and procedure to the patient and the stone. Not all stones need to be treated, but those that do should have the right procedure in a timely manner.

Follow-up after stone treatment is needed to assess for the presence of any residual fragments (RF) that remain after intervention (and to determine whether observation or further active treatment is required), and to identify future issues such as recurrent stone formation and silent obstruction (either as a consequence of instrumentation or recurrent stone formation). In this regard, attention to the imaging modality used is important, to reduce the risk of excessive radiation exposure.

Residual Fragments After ESWL, URS, FURS and PCNL

As far as post ESWL fragments are concerned, the natural history for those ≤4 mm is that 33% of patients become stone free, 29% have stable stones and in 37% they grow after a median follow-up of 40 months. More than 20% of patients need an auxiliary treatment, the majority of which is further ESWL [31]. With fragments ≤4 mm, and a mean follow-up 4.9 years, 78.6% pass spontaneously in few weeks, leaving 21.4% of patients who have regrowth of stones requiring further treatment [32].

More recent data have shown that, in patients with residual fragments after ESWL

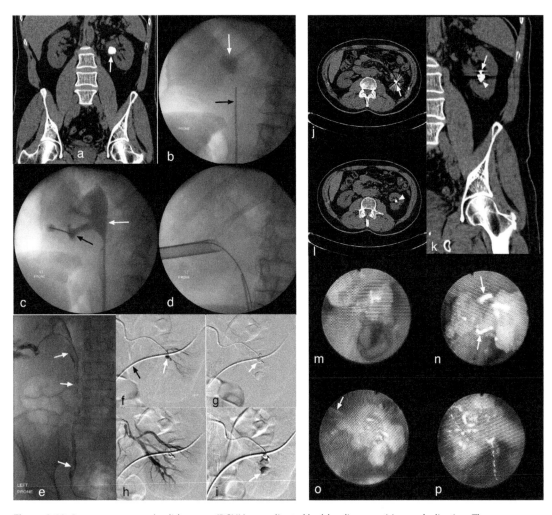

Figure 3.10 Percutaneous nephrolithotomy (PCNL) complicated by bleeding requiring embolisation. These images show a large stone in the left renal pelvis on a coronal CT image (a, arrow), for which a PCNL was performed. The stone is visible (b, white arrow) with a ureteric catheter in position (b, black arrow) in the prone position. Following opacification with contrast, in which the stone is still just visible (c, white arrow) a lower pole puncture (c, black arrow) was performed, with a 30-Fr track via which the stone was fragmented and cleared (d). A nephrostomy was placed postoperatively, with brisk bleeding when it was removed; it was replaced for tamponade and a nephrostogram performed which showed filling defects consistent with blood clots in the renal pelvis and down the ureter (e, arrows).

An angiogram via a selective arterial catheter (f, black arrow) showed a pseudo-aneurysm as the cause of the bleeding (f, white arrow). Embolisation coils are shown (g, arrow) with no further bleeding into the pseudo-aneurysm (h). The last image in this sequence shows contrast in the lower calyx (i, arrow).

The embolisation coils are seen on the axial (j, arrow) and coronal (k, arrow) CT images, performed more than 5 years later, with associated 'beam hardening artefact' and new stone formation (k,l, arrowheads). The stone (k, white arrow) was identified with a flexible ureterorenoscope (m) at which it was evident that the stone had formed on embolisation coils (n, arrows) that had eroded through to the tip of the papilla (onto which the original puncture had been made). The stone was cleared by laser fragmentation (o, arrow) leaving a denuded area with some subepithelial coil still visible where the stone had been attached (p).

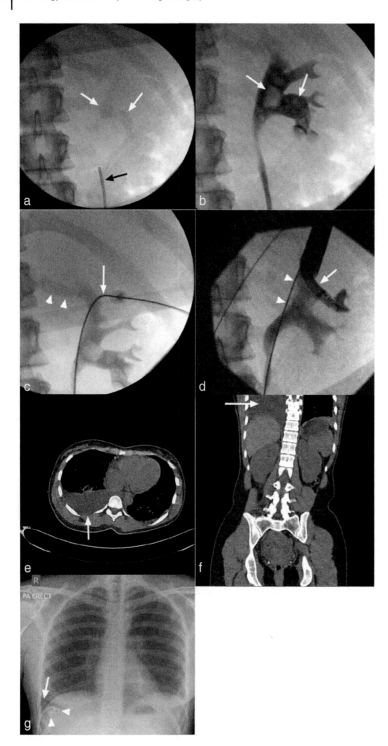

Figure 3.11 PCNL complicated by urothorax requiring chest drain. These images show a patient undergoing a PCNL (prone) for a collection of faintly opaque stones (a, arrows) with a ureteric catheter in position (a, black arrow) that demonstrates multiple stones as filling defects in the renal pelvis and all calyces after contrast is instilled into the collecting system (b, arrows).

A needle puncture and antegrade wire is inserted into the posterior upper pole calyx (c, arrow), noting the presence of a short twelfth rib (c, arrowheads). A suitable track was dilated and secured with an Amplatz® sheath (d, arrowheads) and a flexible nephroscopy (d, white arrow) also passed to minimise the risk of a residual stone. A nephrostomy was placed postoperatively (not shown), with upper abdominal pain and shortness of breath shortly after it was removed. The CT images show a hydrothorax (arrow) in axial (e) and coronal images (f) which resolved rapidly on the insertion of a coiled chest drain. The final image shows the drain in situ (g, arrowheads) with good clearance of the fluid, such that the costo-phrenic angle was visible on chest X-ray (g, arrow) before the drain was uneventfully removed.

stratified by stone size, by 3-month follow-up 52% of fragments >4 mm had passed spontaneously (associated with an accident and emergency department (A&E) visit in about half of the patients), compared with 76% passage for fragments 2–4 mm (with an A&E visit in approximately 20%), with 100% spontaneous passage for fragments ≤2 mm (with no A&E visits) [33].

Broadly similar data are seen with RFs <4 mm following URS, in which 58.7% remained asymptomatic (stable size), 21.7% had spontaneous passage and 19.6% had a 'stone event' (A&E visit or admitted for additional intervention) [34].

In a retrospective analysis of PCNLs performed in 2469 patients, RFs were found in 7.6%, of which the majority was in the lower calix (57.7%), with a mean area of 38.6 ± 52 mm^2. Overall, approximately half of them passed spontaneously, approximately two-thirds within the first 3 months. Stones <25 mm^2 that were located in the renal pelvis had the highest chance of spontaneous passage [35].

Raman *et al.* [36] followed patients with residual fragments (the median size was 2 mm with a range of 1–12 mm) diagnosed on post PCNL CT. 43% of patients had a 'stone-related event' (growth of a residual fragment, symptoms requiring an emergency attendance, hospitalisation or additional intervention) after a median follow-up of 32 months. The need for intervention was predicted by fragments in the renal pelvis or ureter, maximum residual fragment >2 mm and a high cumulative residual fragment size. Overall, 40% of patients with RFs became symptomatic, of whom 40% needed intervention, with 67% of patients with fragments >4 mm becoming symptomatic, of whom 100% needed intervention [36].

The same group made a further analysis, based on a cost comparison between an immediate second look flexible nephroscopy (via the existing PCNL tract) against expectant management. Because of the increased likelihood of symptomatic treatment or further intervention for stones >4 mm, they showed that the average cost of expectant management was $1743 for stones ≤4 mm, compared with $4674 for >4 mm. The additional cost of a second look was $2475, hence a cost advantage for second look procedure for RFs >4 mm [37].

Patients who have embarked on surgery for their stones have a vested interest in achieving clearance. As it is a more invasive treatment, any consequences of RFs after PCNL may be considered more important, because the patient's 'investment' to become stone free is greater. Obstructing fragments require immediate treatment. Whatever the initial modality of treatment, fragments of ≤2 mm are likely to pass with little or no pain. Larger stones, especially within calyces are less likely to pass and more likely to cause symptoms.

If fragments remain at 3 months' follow-up, the patient and surgeon must define for how much longer expectant management can continue. The longer it goes on, the more expensive it becomes and the higher the likelihood of enlargement and symptoms.

Specific recommendations for the timing of follow-up, with what imaging and for what duration before discharging patients from review are difficult owing to the multifactorial nature of stone formation and recurrence. There is also a spectrum of medical complexity in patients, from those in the prime of life who are perfectly fit and well, to those with spina bifida with urinary diversions for intractable bladder complications (perhaps with a solitary kidney).

Stratification of risk is therefore an essential component of follow-up strategy, which begins with the stone analysis and a simple metabolic screen (serum calcium, uric acid, creatinine and estimated glomerular filtration rate). It also includes specific urological anatomical risk factors (e.g. horseshoe kidney, urinary diversion, medullary sponge kidney) and medical risk factors (e.g. hyperparathyroidism, metabolic syndrome, inflammatory bowel disease) (Table 3.2) [38].

The following suggestions are made based on our practice in the stone/endourology

Table 3.2 Risk factors for recurrent stone disease.

Stone	Genetics	Anatomy	Medical conditions	Prior history
Pure calcium oxalate	Primary hyperoxaluria	Calyceal diverticulum	Hyperparathyroidism	Bilateral stones
Pure calcium phosphate (especially brushite – calcium phosphate mono-hydrate)	Renal tubular acidosis	Medullary sponge kidney	Gastrointestinal diseases (jejuno-ileal bypass, intestinal resection, Crohn's disease, malabsorptive conditions, enteric hyperoxaluria after urinary diversion)	Previous rapid stone recurrence (e.g. two stone episodes in 2 years or three in 5 years)
Cystine stone	Cystinuria	Ureteral stricture or ureterocoele	Sarcoidosis	Solitary kidney (does not change risk but increases consequences of recurrence)
Struvite stone		Horseshoe kidney	Nephrocalcinosis	Strong family history
Uric acid stone		PUJ obstruction	Metabolic syndrome	Early age of stone formation

PUJ, pelviureteric junction.
Source: Derived from EAU guidelines and authors' practice [43].

unit at University College Hospitals, London: a post-treatment follow-up to assess for the presence of residual fragments is arranged at 6 weeks, using US which provides more information than plain X-ray (i.e. whether there is hydronephrosis suggesting 'silent obstruction'). The strategy for further follow-up then depends on the size of residual fragments; a simple summary is shown in Figure 3.12.

In general, any stone fragments identified after treatment will behave in the same fashion regardless of the energy source and mode of delivery that created them, and may pass spontaneously (perhaps with an episode of ureteric colic) or remain in situ, where they may cause local discomfort or remain asymptomatic. The latter group needs follow-up to assess for enlargement of the residual stone despite the absence of discomfort, because size is the key determinant for choice of treatment within the kidney, such that ESWL is less likely to be chosen once the stone's maximum diameter has exceeded 10 mm. Patients

who still have symptoms at follow-up should have their stones treated actively, for which the modality is likely to depend on the initial treatment strategy. In particular, if a patient has already had three sessions of ESWL, but still has a stone, the next step is likely to be a 'salvage' ureterorenoscopy. However, if the initial treatment was either FURS or PCNL, with a residual stone <10 mm, the rescue option is likely to be ESWL to achieve clearance without further surgery, although the endourological options should also be discussed.

If the patient is stone free at follow-up, a further review, with timescale adjusted according to the perceived risk of recurrence, would be arranged with KUB US approximately 6–12 months later. At this time, if there has been no recurrence patients can be discharged, or if a concern about recurrence remains, they can be followed up at an increasing time interval. If symptoms occur, the patient should have a route of access between appointments for urgent

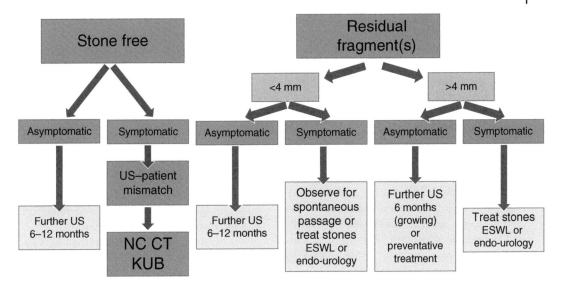

Figure 3.12 A strategy for follow-up after intervention for stone treatment.

reassessment and treatment if needed. In this case, a CT KUB is likely to be the key investigation, either to reassure the patient if 'all clear' or to plan treatment according to the size, location and Hounsfield unit density of any stones found.

Patients who are at high risk should have closer follow-up, and those with significant medical complexity should have a lower threshold for CT follow-up; it is more important to be certain of the stone status in these patients, and there is likely to be less risk of consequence from low dose CT protocols given their co-morbidity. CT is also useful when there is an 'US–patient mismatch' (i.e. no abnormality on US but the patient is symptomatic) or after a long follow-up interval to re-establish the exact stone burden. CT should also be considered before invasive interventions are planned for stones identified on US alone, because US has a tendency to overestimate stone size and therefore the treatment proposed may be more invasive than necessary [39].

Radiation Exposure for Patients with Stones

Patients with nephrolithiasis are at risk from radiation exposure, from their initial diagnostic imaging through the use of fluoroscopy during treatment, and during follow-up (from the surveillance imaging itself and from any additional radiation-based imaging required for the management of recurrent stones). This has become a particular issue because unenhanced CT has established itself as the 'test of choice' for the most accurate evaluation of stone disease [40].

In a 1-year follow-up study of patients after an acute stone episode, the median total effective radiation dose per patient was 29.7 mSv (interquartile range, IQR 24.2–45.1), with 20% receiving a total radiation dose >50 mSv (the recommended yearly dose limit for occupational exposure by the International Commission on Radiological Protection) [41]. Similar first-year exposure was reported by Fahmy *et al.* (29.3 mSv), which decreased to 8.04 mSv (range 1.4–24.72) in the second year, with none exceeding 50 mSv, because of fewer CT scans and more US imaging during the second year [42]. In these studies, the radiation dose did not correlate with stone factors (composition, location or number), patient factors (age and sex) or the surgical intervention performed [41, 42]. In order to minimise the radiation dose, the ALARA ('as low as reasonably achievable') principle of radiation exposure should be followed during intervention using fluoroscopy, particularly in patients undergoing PCNL, who receive an equal or greater amount of radiation during the intervention than during the diagnostic CT beforehand. In this regard, risk factors for increased exposure during PCNL include obesity and a larger stone burden, especially if multiple tracts are used [43].

During ureteroscopy, the fluoroscopic dose is approximately the same as a plain X-ray. Risk factors for increased exposure during ureteroscopy include obesity and performing a ureteric dilatation. Fluoroscopy time during ureteroscopy may be decreased by

a laser-guided C-arm, a dedicated C-arm technician, stent placement under direct vision and tactile feedback to help guide wire placement.

These data indicate that all stone-forming patients are at risk of radiation exposure, including the possibility of receiving a dose >50 mSv, and that this can only be managed by clinician awareness of the imaging modalities being requested. It is advisable to use US as the mainstay of follow-up imaging, and to use 'low dose' CT protocols to provide adequate image quality with reduced radiation exposure compared with standard CT, when this is essential for decision making [40, 44].

References

1 Burgher A, Beman M, Holtzman JL, Monga M. Progression of nephrolithiasis: long-term outcomes with observation of asymptomatic calculi. *J Endourol*. 2004; 18(6): 534–539.

2 Yuruk E, Binbay M, Sari E, *et al.* A prospective, randomized trial of management for asymptomatic lower pole calculi. *J Urol*. 2010; 183(4): 1424–1428.

3 Morse RM, Resnick MI. Ureteral calculi: natural history and treatment in an era of advanced technology. *J Urol*. 1991; 145(2): 263–265.

4 Coll DM, Varanelli MJ, Smith RC. Relationship of spontaneous passage of ureteral calculi to stone size and location as revealed by unenhanced helical CT. *AJR Am J Roentgenol*. 2002; 178(1): 101–103.

5 Holm-Nielsen A, Jørgensen T, Mogensen P, Fogh J. The prognostic value of probe renography in ureteric stone obstruction. *Br J Urol*. 1981; 53(6): 504–507.

6 Irving SO, Calleja R, Lee F, Bullock KN, Wraight P, Doble A. Is the conservative management of ureteric calculi of >4 mm safe? *BJU Int*. 2000; 85(6): 637–640.

7 Seitz C, Fajković H, Remzi M, *et al.* Rapid extracorporeal shock wave lithotripsy

treatment after a first colic episode correlates with accelerated ureteral stone clearance. *Eur Urol*. 2006; 49(6): 1099–1105.

8 Sarica K, Kafkasli A, Yazici Ö, *et al.* Ureteral wall thickness at the impacted ureteral stone site: a critical predictor for success rates after SWL. *Urolithiasis*. 2015; 43(1): 83–88.

9 El-Assmy A, El-Nahas AR, Youssef RF, El-Hefnawy AS, Sheir KZ. Impact of the degree of hydronephrosis on the efficacy of in situ extracorporeal shock-wave lithotripsy for proximal ureteral calculi. *Scand J Urol Nephrol*. 2007; 41(3): 208–213.

10 Pace KT, Weir MJ, Tariq N, Honey RJ. Low success rate of repeat shock wave lithotripsy for ureteral stones after failed initial treatment. *J Urol*. 2000; 164(6): 1905–1907.

11 Shen P, Jiang M, Yang J, *et al.* Use of ureteral stent in extracorporeal shock wave lithotripsy for upper urinary calculi: a systematic review and meta-analysis. *J Urol*. 2011; 186(4): 1328–1335.

12 Perez Castro E, Osther PJ, Jinga V, *et al.* Differences in ureteroscopic stone treatment and outcomes for distal, mid-,

proximal, or multiple ureteral locations: the Clinical Research Office of the Endourological Society ureteroscopy global study. *Eur Urol.* 2014; 66(1): 102–109.

13 Georgescu D, Mulțescu R, Geavlete B, Geavlete P. Intraoperative complications after 8150 semirigid ureteroscopies for ureteral lithiasis: risk analysis and management. *Chirurgia (Bucur).* 2014; 109(3): 369–374.

14 Heers H, Turney BW. Trends in urological stone disease: a 5-year update of Hospital Episode statistics. *BJU Int.* 2016; 118(5): 785–789.

15 El-Nahas AR, El-Tabey NA, Eraky I, *et al.* Semirigid ureteroscopy for ureteral stones: a multivariate analysis of unfavorable results. *J Urol.* 2009; 181(3): 1158–1162.

16 Shields JM, Bird VG, Graves R, Gómez-Marín O. Impact of preoperative ureteral stenting on outcome of ureteroscopic treatment for urinary lithiasis. *J Urol.* 2009; 182(6): 2768–2774.

17 Li H, Na W, Li H, *et al.* Percutaneous nephrolithotomy versus ureteroscopic lithotomy for large (>15 mm) impacted upper ureteral stones in different locations: is the upper border of the fourth lumbar vertebra a good indication for choice of management method? *J Endourol.* 2013; 27(9): 1120–1125.

18 Skolarikos A, Gross AJ, Krebs A, *et al.* Outcomes of Flexible Ureterorenoscopy for Solitary Renal Stones in the CROES URS Global Study. *J Urol.* 2015; 194(1): 137–143.

19 Riley JM, Stearman L, Troxel S. Retrograde ureteroscopy for renal stones larger than 2.5 cm. *J Endourol.* 2009; 23(9): 1395–1398.

20 Traxer O, Thomas A. Prospective evaluation and classification of ureteral wall injuries resulting from insertion of a ureteral access sheath during retrograde intrarenal surgery. *J Urol.* 2013; 189(2): 580–584.

21 Breda A, Ogunyemi O, Leppert JT, Schulam PG. Flexible ureteroscopy and laser lithotripsy for multiple unilateral intrarenal stones. *Eur Urol.* 2009; 55(5): 1190–1196.

22 Alkan E, Avci E, Ozkanli AO, Acar O, Balbay MD. Same-session bilateral retrograde intrarenal surgery for upper urinary system stones: safety and efficacy. *J Endourol.* 2014; 28(7): 757–762.

23 Elbahnasy AM, Shalhav AL, Hoenig DM, *et al.* Lower caliceal stone clearance after shock wave lithotripsy or ureteroscopy: the impact of lower pole radiographic anatomy. *J Urol.* 1998; 159(3): 676–682.

24 Donaldson JF, Lardas M, Scrimgeour D, *et al.* Systematic review and meta-analysis of the clinical effectiveness of shock wave lithotripsy, retrograde intrarenal surgery, and percutaneous nephrolithotomy for lower-pole renal stones. *Eur Urol.* 2015; 67(4): 612–616.

25 Lee SW, Chaiyakunapruk N, Chong HY, Liong ML. Comparative effectiveness and safety of various treatment procedures for lower pole renal calculi: a systematic review and network meta-analysis. *BJU Int.* 2015; 116(2): 252–264.

26 Srisubat A, Potisat S, Lojanapiwat B, Setthawong V, Laopaiboon M. Extracorporeal shock wave lithotripsy (ESWL) versus percutaneous nephrolithotomy (PCNL) or retrograde intrarenal surgery (RIRS) for kidney stones. *Cochrane Database Syst Rev.* 2014; 11: CD007044.

27 Kamphuis GM, Baard J, Westendarp M, de la Rosette JJ. Lessons learned from the CROES percutaneous nephrolithotomy global study. *World J Urol.* 2015; 33(2): 223–233.

28 Singh M, Chapman R, Tresidder GC, Blandy J. The fate of the unoperated staghorn calculus. *Br J Urol.* 1973; 45(6): 581–585.

29 Teichman JM, Long RD, Hulbert JC. Long-term renal fate and prognosis after staghorn calculus management. *J Urol.* 1995; 153(5): 1403–1407.

30 Amer T, Ahmed K, Bultitude M, *et al.* Standard versus tubeless percutaneous nephrolithotomy: a systematic review. *Urol Int.* 2012; 88(4): 373–382.

31 Candau C, Saussine C, Lang H, Roy C, Faure F, Jacqmin D. Natural history of residual renal stone fragments after ESWL. *Eur Urol.* 2000; 37(1): 18–22.

32 Osman MM, Alfano Y, Kamp S, *et al.* 5-year-follow-up of patients with clinically insignificant residual fragments after extracorporeal shockwave lithotripsy. *Eur Urol.* 2005; 47(6): 860–864.

33 Sahin C, Kafkasli A, Cetinel CA, Narter F, Saglam E, Sarica K. How do the residual fragments after SWL affect the health-related quality of life? A critical analysis in a size-based manner. *Urolithiasis.* 2015; 43(2): 163–170.

34 Rebuck DA, Macejko A, Bhalani V, Ramos P, Nadler RB. The natural history of renal stone fragments following ureteroscopy. *Urology.* 2011; 77(3): 564–568.

35 Ganpule A, Desai M. Fate of residual stones after percutaneous nephrolithotomy: a critical analysis. *J Endourol.* 2009; 23(3): 399–403.

36 Raman JD, Bagrodia A, Gupta A, *et al.* Natural history of residual fragments following percutaneous nephrostolithotomy. *J Urol.* 2009; 181(3): 1163–1168.

37 Raman JD, Bagrodia A, Bensalah K, Pearle MS, Lotan Y. Residual fragments after percutaneous nephrolithotomy:

cost comparison of immediate second look flexible nephroscopy versus expectant management. *J Urol.* 2010; 183(1): 188–193.

38 Türk C, Petřík A, Sarica K, *et al.* EAU Guidelines on Interventional Treatment for Urolithiasis. *Eur Urol.* 2016; 69(3): 475–482.

39 Sternberg KM, Eisner B, Larson T, Hernandez N, Han J, Pais VM. Ultrasonography significantly overestimates stone size when compared to low-dose, noncontrast computed tomography. *Urology.* 2016; 95: 67–71.

40 Hyams ES, Shah O. Evaluation and follow-up of patients with urinary lithiasis: minimizing radiation exposure. *Curr Urol Rep.* 2010; 11(2): 80–86.

41 Ferrandino MN, Bagrodia A, Pierre SA, *et al.* Radiation exposure in the acute and short-term management of urolithiasis at two academic centers. *J Urol.* 2009; 181(2): 668–672; discussion 673.

42 Fahmy NM, Elkoushy MA, Andonian S. Effective radiation exposure in evaluation and follow-up of patients with urolithiasis. *Urology.* 2012; 79(1): 43–47.

43 Chen TT, Wang C, Ferrandino MN, *et al.* Radiation exposure during the evaluation and management of nephrolithiasis. *J Urol.* 2015; 194(4): 878–885.

44 Mancini JG, Ferrandino MN. The impact of new methods of imaging on radiation dosage delivered to patients. *Curr Opin Urol.* 2010; 20(2): 163–168.

4

Pelvi-ureteric Junction Reconstruction

Mohamed Ismail and Hash Hashim

Introduction

Pelvi-ureteric junction obstruction (PUJO) is defined as the impairment of urinary transport from the renal pelvis to the upper ureter. Most cases are congenital in origin such as the presence of an aperistaltic segment, true ureteric stricture or the presence of mucosal infolding. However, acquired conditions such as inflammation, stone disease or urothelial malignancy can result in a similar picture [1]. An extrinsic compression caused by an aberrant segmental vessel has recently received much attention as a common cause of PUJO [2].

Antenatal Hydronephrosis

The advent of antenatal ultrasound (US) scanning has led to early diagnosis of the condition. However, mild to moderate hydronephrosis is a common finding in the fetus and may not imply any pathological features. The natural history of the disease remains uncertain. It can prove difficult to distinguish the baby who will have progressive disease because of true obstruction from those who have a variation of normal appearance that will resolve or remain stable.

The majority of infants with antenatally diagnosed PUJO are asymptomatic and the indications for surgical correction remain controversial [3]. The main objective of management is preservation of renal function [4]. Asymptomatic infants with stable renal function can be managed conservatively. Dhillon *et al.* [5] have reported on the Great Ormond Street Hospital (GOSH) experience of conservative management of antenatally detected PUJO. More than half of the patients with dilated kidneys remained stable, one-quarter improved and 17% required surgery. They suggested that the measurement of the anterior–posterior (AP) diameter is a significant predictor for functional impairment. Overall, kidneys with AP diameter >15 mm are more likely to progress and require surgical correction [6].

Heinlen *et al.* [4] reported on the intermediate-term effect of surgical and non-surgical treatment of PUJO in babies. They retrospectively analysed 243 patients with grade 3–4 hydronephrosis on a postnatal US scan (Society of Fetal Urology [SFU] grading). Overall, 48% were found to have obstruction on renogram. Grade of hydronephrosis with parenchymal thinning on ultrasonography and renal function on the renogram determined whether patients would undergo immediate pyeloplasty, pyeloplasty after a period of observation, or observation only. The mean follow-up period was 24 months (3–69 months). In the pyeloplasty group (both immediate and delayed), there was a significant improvement in the

Radiology and Follow-up of Urologic Surgery, First Edition. Edited by Christopher Woodhouse and Alex Kirkham.

differential renal function. In the observation group, the differential renal function stayed stable throughout the follow-up period. In all groups, the degree of hydronephrosis had significantly improved by at least one grade.

Recently, there have been concerns about loss of relative function during conservative management. Babu *et al.* [7] compared the functional outcome 1 year following immediate versus delayed pyeloplasty in patients with antenatally diagnosed unilateral PUJO. Criteria that were used to define significant obstruction included deterioration in split renal function of more than 10%, urine infection or pain. In the delayed pyeloplasty group, 80% suffered loss of split function during a mean follow-up period of 12 months. Delayed surgery was associated with a marginal improvement in split renal function postoperatively but not to baseline levels. Immediate pyeloplasty resulted in a significant improvement in renal function.

In a systematic review of functional outcomes of pyeloplasty in children, it was demonstrated that pyeloplasty is followed by improvement in hydronephrosis and urinary excretion pattern in up to 95% of patients. However, recovery of renal function was much more variable [8]. Babies with initial differential renal function of less than 40% and especially those between 30% and 39% are likely to gain 5–10% (H.K. Dhillon, personal communication 2016, unpublished data quoted with permission).

On GOSH data, about half of all babies managed conservatively will have complete resolution of hydronephrosis. Twenty per cent of babies have hydronephrosis that does not resolve but have no evidence of obstruction and have stable renal function. There is complete follow-up on these patients to 16 years, and in some cases up to 28 years, without any change (H.K. Dhillon, personal communication 2016, unpublished data quoted with permission). Both of these groups should be considered as having a variation of normal that does not require surgery.

Pathophysiological Effect of True Pelvi-ureteric Obstruction

Two distinct histological features of congenital PUJO were described by Hanna *et al.* [9]: excessive collagenosis and compromised muscle cells. In a more recent study, five histological features were described: normal tissue, chronic inflammatory response, smooth muscle hypertrophy, smooth muscle atrophy and fibrosis [2]. Normal ureteric tissue was found in 33% of specimens and was more prominent in the specimens with crossing vessels. Smooth muscle hypertrophy was found in 15% and smooth muscular atrophy in 28%. Chronic inflammation and fibrosis were identified in 37% and 28%, respectively.

Lennon *et al.* [10] investigated the pathophysiological effects of ureteric obstruction. They created an in vivo model of complete and partial ureteric obstruction in dogs. *Complete* ureteric obstruction resulted in total loss of peristaltic movement and was associated with a significant rise in intrarenal and intraureteric pressures. Following relief of obstruction, the contractility pattern returned to baseline but pressure remained high. *Partial* ureteric obstruction was associated with an increase in the contractility amplitude and intrarenal pressure. Eight weeks following the relief of partial obstruction, increased contractility persisted. Renal blood flow increased after ureteric obstruction as a result of decrease in the afferent arteriolar vascular resistance. If obstruction persisted, renal blood flow decreased to 50% of baseline because of an increase in the afferent arteriolar resistance [11]. Glomerular filtration rate (GFR) was initially maintained at 80% of the normal level because of a rise in glomerular filtration pressure and glomerular plasma flow. After 24 hours, GFR was reduced to approximately 30% of the normal level secondary to afferent arteriolar vasoconstriction [12].

Rise in the intrarenal pressure and impaired ureteric contractility leads to urinary pooling giving rise to hydronephrosis. Intratubular urinary pooling causes desquamation and mechanical injury of the tubular epithelium. The final result is the induction of pro-inflammatory and pro-fibrotic reaction leading to tubulointerstitial fibrosis and decreased function [13].

Physiological and Anatomical Changes in the Kidney Following Pyeloplasty

The natural history of PUJO is not clearly defined. Therefore it is difficult to determine which patients will obtain functional benefit from surgical correction. Pyeloplasty is associated with a greater than 95% success rate in relieving the symptoms in those patients who are symptomatic and in preserving renal function [14]. Various radiological modalities have been used post-pyeloplasty, such as US, intravenous pyelogram, CT scan, MAG3 renography and dynamic contrast enhanced magnetic resonance urography (Figures 4.1, 4.2 and 4.3). Serial US and MAG3 renogram are the most commonly used methods to assess the renal unit post pyeloplasty. Surgical success is based on US improvement of

pyelocaliectasis and improved drainage on diuretic renography; in addition to recovery of split renal function and improved symptoms.

Amling [15] has studied the long-term renal US changes after pyeloplasty in children with PUJO. US scans were the same or worse than pre-operative ones during the first month following treatment in 92% of children. At 6 months, 38% had improved. It took 2 years for the pyelocaliectasis to improve in 81% of patients. Ultimately, only 9 of 47 kidneys achieved grade 0 or 1 dilatation (19%) from the grade 3 or 4 that they were pre-operatively (SFU grading) despite renographic confirmation of relief of obstruction. The degree of resolution of hydronephrosis was not related to the pre-operative grade of hydronephrosis [15]. Tapia and Gonzalez [16] have described a reduction in the grade of hydronephrosis in 95% of renal units at 6–12 months. Another study noted an improved or stable hydronephrosis on 3-month postoperative scan [17]. The routine use of JJ stent post pyeloplasty has resulted in improved hydronephrosis in 90% of patients at 1 year follow-up [18]. Overall, pyeloplasty is associated with US downgrading in the level of hydronephrosis in almost all patients [18].

Figure 4.1 Ultrasound (US) showing the classic appearance of the kidney with pelvi-ureteric obstruction (PUJO). The calyces are dilated and the parenchyma thinned. PUJO cannot be diagnosed from this image alone; non-visualisation of the ureter would make it a likely diagnosis.

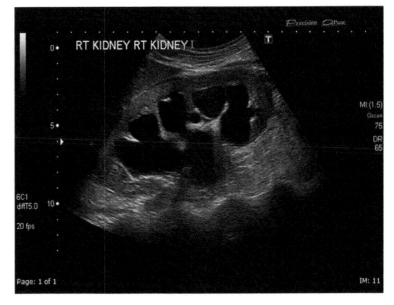

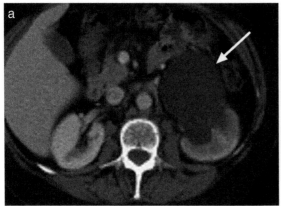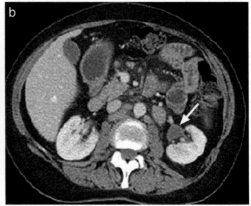

Figure 4.2 (a) CT scan of an adult with left PUJ obstruction (arrow). The renal pelvis is greatly dilated and cortical enhancement delayed. Although this woman had typical obstructive symptoms confirmed on MAG3, the parenchyma is well preserved. (b) CT of the same patient after Anderson–Hynes pyeloplasty. The renal pelvis (arrow) is now of almost normal size, no calyces are visible and the enhancement is symmetrical.

There is not necessarily a direct correlation between improved US features post pyeloplasty and improved renal function. The majority of patients with improved hydronephrosis post pyeloplasty will have stable function on MAG3 renogram but few will have improved function as judged by GFR [17]. Interestingly, the maximum concentrating ability, which is impaired pre-operatively, improves postoperatively in all patients but not to normal levels [19].

Pre-operative renography is essential to confirm the diagnosis and to assess residual renal function. Whether the kidney will recover or retain its pre-operative function may have more to do with the pre-operative renal function than the renogram findings [17]. The role of MAG3 renogram post pyeloplasty follow-up has been a matter of debate. Almodhen *et al.* [20] showed that post-pyeloplasty diuretic renography consistently showed improved drainage. Patients with pre-operative split function of less than 45% demonstrated functional improvement of more than 5% by postoperative renography. Delayed pyeloplasty following a period of observation had a negative impact on split renal function [21].

Historically, serial diuretic renography has been used for long-term postoperative follow-up. However, it has been clearly shown that it is unnecessary if the initial postoperative renogram is non-obstructive [22–24]. Recent literature has questioned whether even the initial postoperative renogram should be routinely performed [20]. It has also been shown that a postoperative renogram is not needed in patients in whom postoperative US revealed improved hydronephrosis. There is only a 2% chance of having postoperative obstructive renography if there is an improvement on US. However, even these were transient and improved with time [20].

Magnetic resonance urography (MRU) has been used to evaluate the anatomy and function of the renal unit post pyeloplasty. MRU was performed pre- and 4 weeks post pyeloplasty. Renal length, renal transit time, renal pelvis AP diameter, differential renal function and single kidney GFR index were calculated [25]. Decreased enhancement, delayed contrast material excretion, swirling contrast medium and contrast urine fluid level in the renal pelvis are signs of obstruction. Postoperatively, the mean AP diameter, differential function and single kidney GFR had all significantly improved. Renal transit time showed a significant drop from 16.2 to 8.6 minutes. MRU provides higher quality

Figure 4.3 MAG3 diuretic renogram of a patient with right PUJO (a) before and (b) after pyeloplasty. The continuously rising curve in the pre-operative picture (ringed) is characteristic of obstruction. The static images show prolonged retention of isotope to the end of the study. Postoperatively, the right renal curve is concave. The static images still show slower clearance than on the left but improved. Even with complete removal of obstruction, isotope clearance is seldom as rapid as on the normal side.

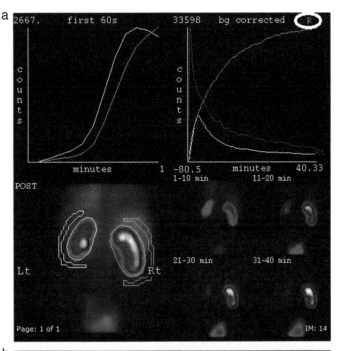

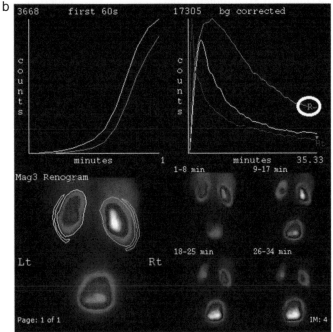

anatomical and functional information to evaluate patients post pyeloplasty; however, higher cost than US and MAG3 renogram remains a major obstacle and it is not necessary for routine use.

Incidental PUJO in adults

A number of PUJO cases are clinically silent in childhood and manifest symptoms in adults. Some can be an incidental finding on routine imaging. The cause of PUJO detected in adulthood is poorly understood. Considering the embryological cause of PUJO, it remains unclear how the kidney survived obstruction over years without losing function. It is also difficult to understand how the patient remains asymptomatic with an obstructed kidney. This could be because of intermittent or incomplete obstruction that preserved the kidney function and hence an asymptomatic patient. The change in the peristaltic pattern found in the partially obstructed dog ureter during induced dieresis could be a cause if applicable to humans. The contractions are of higher than normal pressure (although lower than at normal urine flow rates), are of significantly longer duration and irregular in frequency [10]. The 'binge' drinking associated with young adulthood might change a low grade but safe obstruction into a significant and intermittently symptomatic one.

Many patients present with vague intermittent symptoms and may undergo several tests with inconclusive results. There are very few reports of long-term follow-up of asymptomatic adults with PUJO, mainly because of the reluctance of asymptomatic patients to undergo physiological and radiological investigations.

Kinn [26] has reported on the long-term follow-up of hydronephrosis caused by PUJO in patients who are managed with pyeloplasty or conservative management. Out of 83 patients, 36 were managed conservatively for a mean follow-up of 17 years. In the absence of infection or stone formation, PUJO followed a benign course with no need for surgical intervention. The study revealed that recurrent flank pain was the best indicator of the need for surgery.

The symptomatic patient with an equivocal MAG3 renogram represents a challenging clinical scenario. In a retrospective study, 23 patients with variable flank symptoms were found to have equivocal diuretic renograms defined as a half-life of less than 20 minutes. Minimally invasive pyeloplasty provided symptomatic relief in 22 [27].

In conclusion, if the patient is asymptomatic with stable overall and split renal function, conservative management with serial imaging may be appropriate. The indications of intervention for PUJO detected later in life include symptoms, impaired renal function and the development of renal stones or recurrent infection. If we look at the trends in management of adults with PUJO, most patients will undergo minimally invasive pyeloplasty and this explains the scarcity of literature on the long-term outcome of conservative management of PUJO in adults [28].

Long-term Follow-up

There are no guidelines on the best follow-up protocol for patients after pyeloplasty. Several regimes have been reported based on the 'expert opinion' of the authors [22, 29–31]. None have high level evidence to support them and all seem to be unnecessarily intense.

The aims are slightly different for children and adults. However, in both there is ample evidence that a successful pyeloplasty is a cure for obstruction at the pelvi-ureteric junction. The only question, therefore, is what constitutes success? It should be clear from the outcomes already discussed that elimination of symptoms is the best marker of success. As an objective measure, any improvement in the degree of dilatation of the calyces on ultrasound indicates that obstruction has been relieved. As the dilatation at 3 months is likely to be unchanged or worse, the first ultrasound should be carried out at 6 months. It should be repeated at 6-monthly intervals until there is improvement. MAG3 renogram should only be carried out for symptoms or failure to improve after 2 years. As pyeloplasty produces no significant improvement in renal function, there is no point in measuring serum creatinine unless the condition is bilateral. In patients operated in childhood, the cure is maintained at least up to 5.5 years and to 18 years in those diagnosed antenatally, follow-up that seems long enough to be definitive [32]. Overall obstruction recurred 8 years postoperatively in 0.8% [22]. Although bizarre case reports can be found in the literature, there are no long-term complications directly related to PUJO repair except where there has been such severe damage that renal failure ensues.

Children often are asymptomatic, especially when diagnosed in utero, and the aim of follow-up is to exclude persistent silent obstruction that damages the kidney. Therefore, more intensive long-term follow-up in the paediatric group may be justified. However, it must also be noted that follow-up of any patient, but especially children, generates its own problems. The implication is that there is a 'disease' or that one might develop in the future. This is a cause of anxiety for the family. In adult life it may cause social problems such as loading of insurance premiums because the patient has not had a 'curative' procedure [33].

Several clinical units have guidelines for the follow-up of antenatally diagnosed hydronephrosis with a normal ureter. The most comprehensive at present is from the National Center for Biotechnological Information (NCBI) [34]. Unfortunately, the recommendations on cessation of follow-up are incomplete. After delivery, the first reliable US is at 4–6 weeks (before that time relative dehydration may obscure significant dilatation). If this examination is normal, the baby should be discharged. In these guidelines, the finding of an AP diameter >10 mm is an indication for renogram. Obstructed drainage and differential function of the affected kidney below 35–40% is an indication for surgery. The operation should be curative and the baby can then be discharged as with symptomatic PUJO.

Between these two extremes there are children whose dilatation will completely resolve or at least remain stable, and others who whose kidney will slowly deteriorate and require later surgery. On SFU criteria, at least 90% of those with grade 1 disease will resolve and virtually none will require

surgery. About 75% of grade 3 and all of grade 4 will have had surgery by 7 years or 10 years at the latest. To date, in the GOSH series, no child with an AP diameter of <25 mm has required surgery (H.K. Dhillon, personal communication 2016, unpublished data quoted with permission).

The guidelines recommend that those with grade 1 and 2 should have ultrasounds every 3–6 months until 2 years old and every 6–12 months until resolution or to 6 years old. The unstated implication is that those whose kidney has remained dilated can also be discharged.

Expert opinion is quoted to recommend 'close surveillance' of children with grade 3 or 4 dilatation but without defining means or intervals. There seems little point in performing an ultrasound more often than 3-monthly – if the doctor is that worried, it would probably be better to operate. Diuretic renography is recommended at 6–8 weeks of age and then 3–6 monthly if the US appearances deteriorate.

In bilateral cases with grade 1 and 2, the same criteria for monitoring are recommended. However, as the differential function on renography cannot be used, more attention has to be paid to the pattern of isotope clearance and to measurement of total renal function.

Conclusions

Patients with hydrocalycosis and a normal ureter do not necessarily have obstruction. They can now be divided into two clinical groups: those who are identified in utero, many of whom do not have obstruction, and those found after birth with or without symptoms, most of whom are obstructed. The former group must be subdivided after birth into those who are obstructed and need surgery, those who are not obstructed but have a variation of normality and those who are equivocal.

All patients who are obstructed, in whichever group, should have a pyeloplasty which should be curative. They should be discharged as soon as cure of obstruction is confirmed unless there are other co-morbidities that require monitoring. In the antenatally diagnosed group, those managed conservatively should be discharged as soon as absence of obstruction is established which may be as early a few months, but no later than 6 years. Monitoring of those in the equivocal group should establish whether surgery is needed before the age of 10 but preferably before 7 years old.

References

1 Anderson KR, Weiss RM. Physiology and evaluation of ureteropelvic junction obstruction. *J Endourol*. 1996; 10(2): 87–91.

2 Richstone L, Seideman CA, Reggio E, *et al.* Pathologic findings in patients with ureteropelvic junction obstruction and crossing vessels. *Urology*. 2009; 73(4): 716–719; discussion 719.

3 Gurbuz C, Best SL, Donnally C, Mir S, Pearle MS, Cadeddu JA. Intermediate term outcomes associated with the surveillance of ureteropelvic junction obstruction in adults. *J Urol*. 2011; 185(3): 926–929.

4 Heinlen JE, Manatt CS, Bright BC, Kropp BP, Campbell JB, Frimberger D. Operative versus nonoperative management of ureteropelvic junction obstruction in children. *Urology*. 2009; 73(3): 521–525; discussion 525.

5 Dhillon J. Prenatally diagnosed hydronephrosis: the Great Ormond Street experience. *Br J Urol*. 1998; 81(Suppl 2): 39–44.

6 Hothi DK, Wade AS, Gilbert R, Winyard PJD. Mild fetal renal pelvis dilatation: much ado about nothing? *Clin J Am Soc Nephrol* 2009; 4(1): 168–177.

7 Babu R, Rathish VR, Sai V. Functional outcomes of early versus delayed pyeloplasty in prenatally diagnosed pelvi-ureteric junction obstruction. *J Pediatr Urol*. 2015; 11(2): 63.e1–63.e5.

8 Castagnetti M, Novara G, Beniamin F, Vezzú B, Rigamonti W, Artibani W. Scintigraphic renal function after unilateral pyeloplasty in children: a systematic review. *Br J Urol Int*. 2008; 102(7): 862–868.

9 Hanna MK, Jeffs RD, Sturgess JM, Barkin M. Ureteral structure and ultrastructure. Part II. Congenital ureteropelvic junction obstruction and primary obstructive megaureter. *J Urol*. 1976; 116(6): 725–730.

10 Lennon GM, Ryan PC, Fitzpatrick JM. Recovery of ureteric motility following complete and partial ureteric obstruction. *Br J Urol*. 1993; 72(5 Pt 2): 702–707.

11 Wilson DR. Pathophysiology of obstructive nephropathy. *Kidney Int*. 1980; 18(3): 281–292.

12 Dal Canton A, Corradi A, Stanziale R, Maruccio G, Migone L. Effects of 24-hour unilateral ureteral obstruction on glomerular hemodynamics in rat kidney. *Kidney Int*. 1979; 15(5): 457–462.

13 Mundy AR. *The Scientific Basis of Urology*, 3rd edn. London: Informa Healthcare; 2010.

14 Hashim H, Woodhouse CRJ. Ureteropelvic junction obstruction. *Eur Urol Suppl*. 2012; 11(2): 25–32.

15 Amling CL, O'Hara SM, Wiener JS, Schaeffer CS, King LR. Renal ultrasound changes after pyeloplasty in children with ureteropelvic junction obstruction: long-term outcome in 47 renal units. *J Urol*. 1996; 156(6): 2020–2024.

16 Tapia J, Gonzalez R. Pyeloplasty improves renal function and somatic growth in children with ureteropelvic junction obstruction. *J Urol*. 1995; 154(1): 218–222.

17 Cost NG, Prieto JC, Wilcox DT. Screening ultrasound in follow-up after pediatric pyeloplasty. *Urology*. 2010; 76(1): 175–179.

18 Egan SC, Stock JA, Hanna MK. Renal ultrasound changes after internal double-J stented pyeloplasty for ureteropelvic junction obstruction. *Tech Urol*. 2001; 7(4): 276–280.

19 Bratt CG, Aurell M, Jonsson O, Nilsson S. Long-term followup of maximum concentrating ability and glomerular filtration rate in adult obstructed kidneys after pyeloplasty. *J Urol*. 1988; 140(2): 273–276.

20 Almodhen F, Jednak R, Capolicchio JP, Eassa W, Brzezinski A, El-Sherbiny M. Is routine renography required after pyeloplasty? *J Urol*. 2010; 184(3): 1128–1133.

21 McAleer IM, Kaplan GW. Renal function before and after pyeloplasty: does it improve? *J Urol*. 1999; 162(3, Pt 2): 1041–1044.

22 Psooy K, Pike JG, Leonard MP. Long-term followup of pediatric dismembered pyeloplasty: how long is long enough? *J Urol*. 2003; 169(5): 1809–1812; discussion 1812; author reply 1812.

23 van den Hoek J, de Jong A, Scheepe J, van der Toorn F, Wolffenbuttel K. Prolonged follow-up after paediatric pyeloplasty: are repeat scans necessary? *Br J Urol Int*. 2007; 100(5): 1150–1152.

24 Pohl HG, Rushton HG, Park JS, Belman AB, Majd M. Early diuresis renogram findings predict success following pyeloplasty. *J Urol*. 2001; 165(6 Pt 2): 2311–2315.

25 Kirsch AJ, McMann LP, Jones RA, Smith EA, Scherz HC, Grattan-Smith JD. Magnetic resonance urography for evaluating outcomes after pediatric pyeloplasty. *J Urol*. 2006; 176(4 Pt 2): 1755–1761.

26 Kinn AC. Ureteropelvic junction obstruction. Long-term followup of adults with and without surgical treatment. *J Urol*. 2000; 164(3, Pt 1): 652–656.

27 Ozayar A, Friedlander JI, Shakir NA, Gahan JC, Cadeddu JA, Morgan MS. Equivocal ureteropelvic junction obstruction on diuretic renogram: should minimally invasive pyeloplasty be offered to symptomatic patients? *J Urol*. 2015; 193(4): 1278–1282.

28 Jacobs BL, Kaufman SR, Morgenstern H, Hollenbeck BK, Wolf JS, Hollingsworth JM. Trends in the treatment of adults with ureteropelvic junction obstruction. *J Endourol*. 2013; 27(3): 355–360.

29 O'Reilly PH, Brooman PJ, Mak S, *et al*. The long-term results of Anderson–Hynes pyeloplasty. *Br J Urol Int*. 2001; 87(4): 287–289.

30 Seo IY, Oh TH, Lee JW. Long-term follow-up results of laparoscopic pyeloplasty. *Korean J Urol*. 2014; 55(10): 656–659.

31 Notley RG, Beaugie JM. The long-term follow-up of Anderson–Hynes pyeloplasty for hydronephrosis. *Br J Urol*. 1973; 45(5): 464–467.

32 Chertin B, Pollack A, Koulikov D, *et al*. Does renal function remain stable after puberty in children with prenatal hydronephrosis and improved renal function after pyeloplasty? *J Urol*. 2009; 182 (4 Suppl): 1845–1848.

33 LaSalle MD, Stock JA, Hanna MK. Insurability of children with congenital urological anomalies. *J Urol*. 1997; 158(3 Pt 2): 1312–1315.

34 Sinha A, Bagga A, Krishna A, *et al*. Revised guidelines on management of antenatal hydronephrosis. *Indian J Neprol*. 2013; 23(2): 83–79.

5

Retroperitoneal Fibrosis

Paul Scheel and Bruce Berlanstein

Introduction

Retroperitoneal fibrosis (RPF) is a condition characterised by the presence of inflammation and fibrosis in the retroperitoneal space. Unfortunately, there is no standard definition that clearly defines the criteria that must be present for a diagnosis of RPF. It is this ambiguity that has made formal investigation into the disease challenging and comparison of multiple different reports vulnerable to misinterpretation. As a starting point, most agree that a pathological specimen obtained anywhere in the retroperitoneum indicating fibrosis is not sufficient for the diagnosis of RPF. Rather, the salient feature that must be present is the radiographic finding of a soft tissue density surrounding the infra-renal aorta or proximal iliacs (peri-aortitis). There are currently five diseases that lead to infra-renal peri-aortitis: RPF; inflammatory abdominal aortic aneurysm (IAAA); peri-aneurysmal retroperitoneal fibrosis, Erdheim–Chester disease (ECD), and immunoglobulin 4 (IgG-4)-related disease. In most reports, IAAA and peri-aneurysmal retroperitoneal fibrosis have been lumped together for the purposes of analysis. ECD, while sharing some similar radiographic features, has a distinct histological and clinical presentation. IgG4-related disease was not recognised as a possible isolated condition until 2003. It is unclear how many, if any, of these patients were included in analysis of patients with RPF. Because no standard definition exists, it is important to establish the definition to be used when discussing patients treated for RPF. The following criteria must be present:

1 A soft tissue density surrounding the infra-renal aorta or iliac vessels by contrast-enhanced computed tomography (CT) or magnetic resonance imaging (MRI) (Figures 5.1 and 5.2);
2 Absence of a biopsy that is positive for malignancy;
3 Absence of a systemic multicentric fibrosing process such as IgG4-related disease.

Available Treatments

Medical Therapy

Inflammation is the inciting event in RPF. If left untreated, this fibro-inflammatory process will lead to ureteric obstruction, and obstruction of key vascular structures such as the inferior vena cava, renal vessels or iliac vessels (Figures 5.3, 5.4 and 5.5) [1–4]. Therefore, the goals of therapy are to halt inflammation, reverse fibrosis and implement measures to protect the kidney from chronic injury from ureteric obstruction [5]. It is important for the treating urologist to understand which medical therapy was a utilized when assessing a patient for

Radiology and Follow-up of Urologic Surgery, First Edition. Edited by Christopher Woodhouse and Alex Kirkham.
© 2018 John Wiley & Sons Ltd. Published 2018 by John Wiley & Sons Ltd.

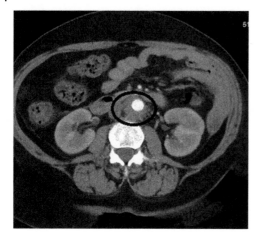

Figure 5.1 Computed tomography (CT) scan of the abdomen with intravenous contrast. There is a soft tissue mass surrounding the infra-renal aorta (ringed).

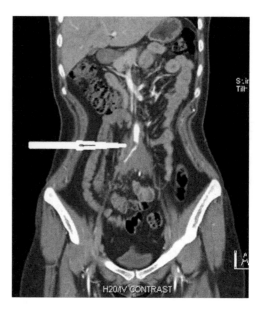

Figure 5.3 CT scan of the pelvis with intravenous contrast. There is significant narrowing of the common iliac artery on the right secondary to extrinsic compression from retroperitoneal fibrosis (RPF; arrow).

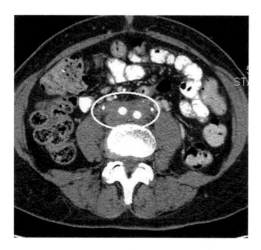

Figure 5.2 CT scan of the pelvis with intravenous contrast. Note soft tissue density surrounding the iliac arteries (ringed).

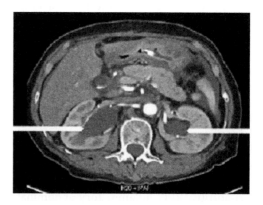

Figure 5.4 CT scan of abdomen with intravenous contrast. Note bilateral (R>L) proximal hydroureter (arrows).

potential ureterolysis as an alternative to failed medical therapy as rates of success and relapse differ significantly [6, 7].

There is no one immunosuppressive protocol that has been shown to be superior to other treatment options. The immunosuppressive therapies that have the most data include corticosteroids, tamoxifen and mycophenolate mofetil (MMF). The only randomised controlled trial (RCT) for the

treatment of RPF was conducted by Vaglio *et al.* [6]. In this small trial, 36 patients with RPF were randomised to treatment with steroids alone or steroids plus tamoxifen. At the start of treatment all patients received prednisone 1 mg/kg/day. After 1 month, or when patients achieved a clinical remission, they were randomised to a prednisone taper

Figure 5.5 Magnetic resonance (MR) venogram of the abdomen. Note lack of contrast in the inferior vena cava (IVC) with narrowing (between lines).

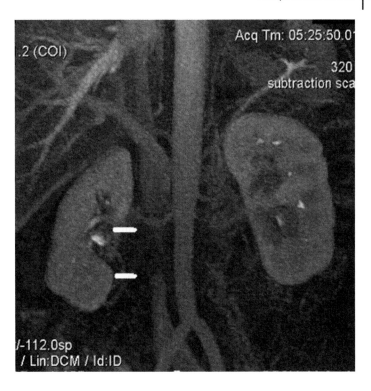

over 7 months or 7 months of tamoxifen. Six per cent of patients in the steroid arm and 39% of patients in the tamoxifen arm relapsed during therapy. Following discontinuation of therapy, the steroid group had an 11.8% relapse rate and the tamoxifen arm had an 18.2% relapse rate. There was no difference in the time to removal of ureteric stents in those patients who had obstructed ureters and there was a greater reduction in the peri-aortic mass in the steroid group.

MMF combined with low dose steroids has been shown to be effective in a prospective series. MMF is an inosine monophosphate inhibitor that interrupts the immune response of T and B cells. In addition, MMF has been shown to reverse fibrosis in laboratory animals [8–10].

Scheel *et al.* [7] initially reported on 28 patients with RPF treated with MMF and low dose steroids. The treatment consisted of oral prednisone 40 mg administered for 30 days with a 10-mg taper each month combined with MMF 1 g administered orally twice daily. The MMF was continued for 6 months following resolution of ureteric obstruction. For patients without ureteric obstruction, the drug was continued for 6 months following a 25% reduction in the peri-aortic mass and complete resolution of symptoms. Patients were treated for a mean of 29.3 months. Eighty per cent of patients had a >25% reduction in the peri-aortic mass and 86% of patients with obstruction had successful removal of ureteric stent(s). Only 7% of patients in this series relapsed. This series has now expanded to over 220 patients with a treatment success rate of 95% and a 5% relapse rate (unpublished data).

Surgical Treatment

Because of the success of medical therapy in reducing the inflammation, size of the peri-aortic mass and eventual extubation of the ureters, there has been a recent paradigm shift toward medical therapy for RPF. The indications for surgery are now reserved for those patients:

1 Who fail medical therapy;
2 Who are unwilling to proceed with a prolonged course of immunosuppressive therapy and repeated stent exchanges;
3 With a contraindication to immunosuppressive therapy such as active bacterial or viral infection.

Surgery can be performed through an open laparotomy, laparoscopic or robotic-assisted technique [11–15]. The goal of ureterolysis is to move the ureter to a more lateral position with both 'intraperitonealisation' and/ or omental wrapping, with a goal of moving the ureter sufficiently out of harm's way of the ongoing inflammation. Follow-up imaging will show a laterally displaced ureter that may or may not have radiographic evidence of continued upper tract dilatation (Figure 5.6). For these patients it is important to document adequate drainage with a MAG3 nuclear medicine renogram or via Whitaker manometry. While these techniques allow for rapid extubation of the affected ureter, a surgical approach fails to treat the underlying ongoing inflammation with associated morbidities of weight loss, pain, anaemia and continued deposition of additional fibrosis.

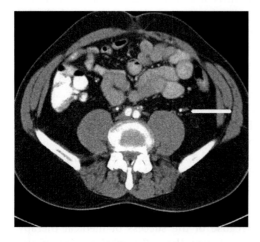

Figure 5.6 CT scan of the abdomen with intravenous contrast in a patient following left ureterolysis for RPF. Note lateral displacement of left ureter (arrow).

Follow-up

Imaging

For patients treated medically, most protocols report cross-sectional imaging every 4–6 months. For those patients with a serum creatinine level of <1.5 mg/dL (132.6 µmol/L), our protocol includes CT of the abdomen and pelvis with possible arterial, venous and urogram (delayed) images. The diameter of the peri-aortic soft tissue mass is best evaluated during the arterial phase images (Figure 5.7). For those patients with disease surrounding the iliac vessels, arterial and venous phase images can be important when discerning if the inflammatory mass continues to affect the ipsilateral stented ureter (Figure 5.8). For those patients who do not have bilateral ureteric stents, we also include urogram images to assess for patency of the unstented ureter.

Stent Removal

For those patients with unilateral or bilateral stents where cross-sectional imaging demonstrates a reduction of the peri-aortic or peri-iliac mass and where the affected ureter(s) is free from the fibro-inflammatory density, we suggest removal of one stent at a time.

Following removal, our patients are assessed for increased pain and decreased urine output. At 48 hours, blood is obtained for analysis of creatinine and potassium levels. If there is no clinical suspicion of obstruction, a MAG3 scan with furosemide washout is obtained at 14 days. If excretion is normal (T-1/2 excretion of less than 12 minutes), one proceeds with removal of a contralateral stent with a similar protocol. At this 14-day stage, a partial obstruction may exist, owing to ureteric oedema associated with prolonged ureteric intubation. If a partial obstruction is demonstrated at day 14 (T-1/2 excretion of 12–20 minutes), the examination is repeated in 2 weeks. If a partial obstruction still exists, the ureteric stent is replaced. If the follow-up study indicates no obstruction, the stent can

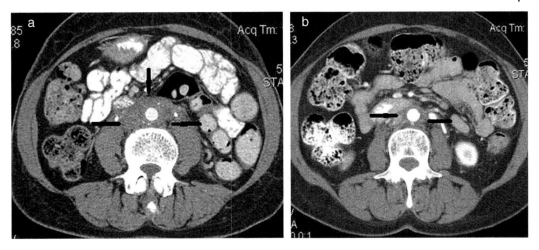

Figure 5.7 CT scan of abdomen with intravenous contrast: (a) before and (b) after medical therapy. Note reduction in size of peri-aortic soft tissue mass (arrows).

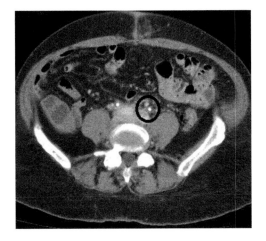

Figure 5.8 CT scan of the pelvis with intravenous contrast. Note ureter crossing left iliac vessels without evidence of obstruction (ringed).

remain out and the contralateral stent, if present, is removed using a similar protocol. For those patients where ureteric obstruction was relieved with a percutaneous nephrostomy (PCN) and where cross-sectional imaging suggests regression of the mass sufficiently to relieve the obstruction, patency can be assessed by closing the external stopcock and proceeding with a MAG3 scan with furosemide washout as described above or by formal Whitaker manometry.

Complications

Stent-related Complications

In all of the aforementioned studies, patients with ureteric obstruction were managed with ureteric stents or PCN tubes until successful reduction in the peri-aortic mass.

Despite the fact that ureteric stents have been used extensively for short-term therapy following treatment of urinary calculi or 'long-term' for palliation of ureteric obstruction with inoperable cancer, few data are available on their optimal management of stents for those patients needing decompression for long periods of time but where the goal is eventual extubation as seen in those patients treated medically with RPF.

Complications from ureteric stents are well known and include the following:

1 Inadequate relief of obstruction;
2 Bladder irritation and pain;
3 Infection;
4 Encrustation and incrustation;
5 Stent fragmentation; and
6 Migration.

Adequate relief of obstruction by extrinsic ureteric compression has been poor and reported to be as low as 40% [16]. Most patients in these series had extrinsic compression secondary to malignancy and very few series have quantified adequate decompression in those patients with RPF. Rosevear *et al.* [17] reported on 20 patients with RPF and reported that 85% patients who were treated with ureteric stents had adequate drainage. In most series, assessment of adequacy of drainage has been limited to those patients who fail to return to baseline creatinine or those with ongoing flank pain post stent placement. Repeat cross-sectional imaging is usually performed every 4–6 months and ongoing hydronephrosis, which suggests poor drainage, would necessitate investigation with MAG3 renography. If an obstruction was confirmed, alternative drainage procedures such as PCN, tandem double J's (JJ)or nephro-ureteric stents (NUS) would be needed [18]. Patients with RPF and ureteric obstruction require stents for 6 months to 3 years. Depending on the study, up to 80% of patients will experience pain, especially with voiding [19]. This pain is independent of stent composition or size but does seem to worsen when the terminal position of the stents in the bladder crosses the midline (Figure 5.9) [20, 21]. As urgency, frequency and significant pain are thought to result from involuntary muscle contractions,

alpha-blockers have been shown to significantly reduce pain in these patients [22–24]. For those patients unable to tolerate JJ stents secondary to significant pain, PCN is the only alternative option for relief of upper tract obstruction.

Incrustation and encrustation of ureteric stents are well-known complications of these devices and can lead to inadequate drainage, difficultly with exchange or removal, as well as stent fracture and migration (Figure 5.10). The degree of encrustation and incrustation is greater in stents less than 6 French and is proportional to duration of time any indwelling stent remains in situ. Kawahara *et al.* [25] reported on 333 stents in 181 patients. In total, 40% of removed stents were encrusted, with 13.9% showing resistance to removal. Twenty six per cent of stents in place for less than 6 weeks were encrusted whereas 56.8% were encrusted if in place for 6–12 weeks rising to 75% for those in place for 12 weeks or longer. In an attempt to balance patient convenience with morbidity, it is for this reason that we suggest changing JJ stents every 3 months.

Ureteric stricture is typically thought of as a reason to place a stent and not as a direct

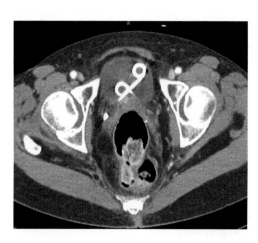

Figure 5.9 CT scan of the pelvis. Note two JJ stents in the bladder with the terminal ends of each stent crossing the midline. Source: Woodhouse 2015 [30], with permission of John Wiley & Sons Ltd.

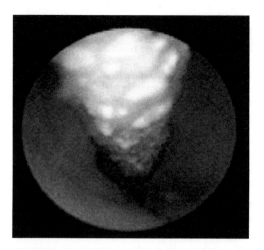

Figure 5.10 Intraoperative photograph taken during ureteroscopy demonstrating encrustation of JJ stent. Picture courtesy of Dr Takashi Kawahara.

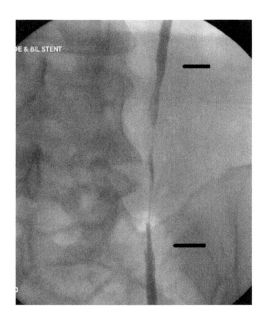

Figure 5.11 Retrograde pyelogram in a patient treated medically for RPF. Note mid ureteric stricture (between arrows). At the time of operative repair, there was no residual evidence of RPF.

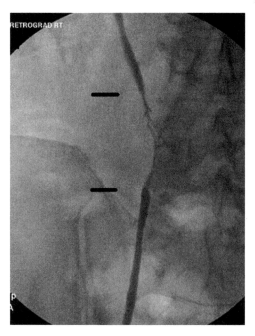

Figure 5.12 Retrograde pyelogram in a patient treated medically for RPF. Note stricture in mid to distal ureter (between arrows). As with the patient in Figure 5.11, there was no residual RPF at surgery. Source: Woodhouse 2015 [30], with permission of John Wiley & Sons Ltd.

result of placement of such devices. Instrumentation of the ureter via ureteroscopy is however a well-documented aetiology of ureteric strictures, occurring in 8–13% of cases [26, 27], and recurrent ureteric instrumentation for stent placementmay also be a cause of stricture formation. Similar to reports of patients with strictures following ureteroscopy, the strictures tend to occur in the mid to distal ureter (Figures 5.11 and 5.12). Strictures should be suspected in those patients with resolution of RPF on cross-sectional imaging but who have evidence of high grade obstruction on MAG3. Strictures can be confirmed by retrograde pyelogram and typically require surgical repair.

Hydrocoeles

Scrotal swelling and pain secondary to hydrocoeles are common in males with RPF and may be a presenting symptom [28]. The pathogenesis is believed to be secondary to interruption of the retroperitoneal lymphatics associated with the fibro-inflammatory process. The incidence in males presenting with RPF has not been formally studied but up to 30% of males presenting to an RPF clinic have a recent diagnosis of a hydrocoele confirmed by ultrasound (US) (Figure 5.13) [29]. Unfortunately, not all of these abnormalities resolve with medical or surgical treatment of the underlying RPF and may need to be addressed with hydrocoelectomy in symptomatic patients.

Long-term Follow-up

RPF has been reported to recur at high rates, depending on the original treatment protocol. This recurrence can occur within

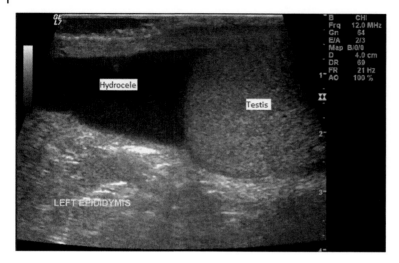

Figure 5.13 Ultrasound scan of the scrotum demonstrating left testicle adjacent to small left hydrocoele.

months to years following discontinuation of immunosuppressive therapy and therefore follow-up must be for the life of the patient. Following discontinuation of immunosuppressive medication, the authors obtained monthly laboratory data assessing for renal function, anaemia and evidence of systemic inflammation (erythrocyte sedimentation rate, ESR; C-reactive protein, CRP) for the first 6 months and every 3 months thereafter. Cross-sectional imaging continues every 6 months for 2 years following discontinuation of medication. Patients are seen twice yearly for 2 years following discontinuation of medical therapy and annually thereafter (Table 5.1). Patients are instructed to contact us immediately if they experience flank pain or unexpected weight loss.

Recurrent Disease

Those patients who have recurrent symptomatic disease (pain, weight loss, increased markers of inflammation or obstruction) associated with recurrent or enlarging peri-aortic or peri-iliac mass are restarted on an immunosuppressive protocol, with or without ureteric stents, similar to de novo patients.

Table 5.1 Suggested protocol for the follow-up of asymptomatic patients who have completed immunosuppressive protocol for retroperitoneal fibrosis. Assumes all ureteric stents have been removed.

Procedure	Follow-up frequency		
	Months 1–6	Months 6–24	Months 24→
Renal profile	Monthly	Every 3 months	Every 3 months
CBC	Monthly	Every 3 months	Every 3 months
ESR	Monthly	Every 3 months	Every 3 months
CRP	Monthly	Every 3 months	Every 3 months
CT or MRI	Month 6	Every 6 months	Prn symptoms
MD visit	Month 6	Every 6 months	Annually

CBC, complete blood count; CRP, C-reactive protein; CT, ESR, erythrocyte sedimentation rate; MD, primary physician; MRI, magnetic resonance imaging; prn, as necessary.

References

1 Haynes IG, Simon J, West RJ, Hamer JD. Idiopathic retroperitoneal fibrosis with occlusion of the abdominal aorta treated by transluminal angioplasty. *Br J Surg.* 1982; 69(7): 432–433.

2 Kerwin G, Silverstein M, Lewis C. Percutaneous stent treatment for arterial occlusion caused by retroperitoneal fibrosis. *AJR Am J Roentgenol.* 2000; 175(5): 1283–1285.

3 Paetzold S, Gary T, Hafner F, Brodmann M. Thrombosis of the inferior vena cava related to Ormond's disease. *Clin Rheumatol.* 2013; 32(Suppl 1): 67–70.

4 Ezimora A, Faulkner ML, Adebiyi O, Ogungbemile A, Marianna SV, Nzerue C. Retroperitoneal fibrosis: a rare cause of acute renal failure. *Case Rep Nephrol.* 2012; 2012: 645407.

5 Scheel PJ Jr, Feeley N. Retroperitoneal fibrosis. *Rheum Dis Clin North Am.* 2013; 39(2): 365–381.

6 Vaglio A, Palmisano A, Alberici F, *et al.* Prednisone versus tamoxifen in patients with idiopathic retroperitoneal fibrosis: an open-label randomised controlled trial. *Lancet.* 2011; 378: 338–346.

7 Scheel PJ Jr, Feeley N, Sozio SM. Combined prednisone and mycophenolate mofetil treatment for retroperitoneal fibrosis: a case series. *Ann Intern Med.* 2011; 154(1): 31–36.

8 Badid C, Vincent M, McGregor B, *et al.* Mycophenolate mofetil reduces myofibroblast infiltration and collagen III deposition in rat remnant kidney. *Kidney Int.* 2000; 58(1): 51–61.

9 Kramer S, Loof T, Martini S, *et al.* Mycophenolate mofetil slows progression in anti-thy1-induced chronic renal fibrosis but is not additive to a high dose of enalapril. *Am J Physiol Renal Physiol.* 2005; 289(2): F359–368.

10 Paz Z, Shoenfeld Y. Antifibrosis: to reverse the irreversible. *Clin Rev Allergy Immunol.* 2010; 38(2–3): 276–286.

11 Carini M, Selli C, Rizzo M, Durval A, Costantini A. Surgical treatment of retroperitoneal fibrosis with omentoplasty. *Surgery.* 1982; 91(2): 137–141.

12 Demirci D, Gülmez I, Ekmekçioğlu O, Sözüer EM, Keklik E. Intraperitonealization of the ureter during laparoscopic ureterolysis: a modification of the technique. *J Urol.* 2001; 165(1): 180–181.

13 Fugita OE, Jarrett TW, Kavoussi P, Kavoussi LR. Laparoscopic treatment of retroperitoneal fibrosis. *J Endourol.* 2002; 16(8): 571–574.

14 Keehn AY, Mufarrij PW, Stifelman MD. Robotic ureterolysis for relief of ureteral obstruction from retroperitoneal fibrosis. *Urology.* 2011; 77(6): 1370–1374.

15 Styn NR, Frauman S, Faerber GJ, Wolf JS Jr., University of Michigan surgical experience with ureterolysis for retroperitoneal fibrosis: a comparison of laparoscopic and open surgical approaches. *Urology.* 2011; 77(2): 339–343.

16 Chung SY, Stein RJ, Landsittel D, *et al.* 15-year experience with the management of extrinsic ureteral obstruction with indwelling ureteral stents. *J Urol.* 2004; 172(2): 592–595.

17 Rosevear HM, Kim SP, Wenzler DL, Faerber GJ, Roberts WW, Wolf JS Jr., Retrograde ureteral stents for extrinsic ureteral obstruction: nine years' experience at University of Michigan. *Urology.* 2007; 70(5): 846–850.

18 Varnavas M, Bolgeri M, Mukhtar S, Anson K. The role of tandem double-J ureteral stents in the management of malignant ureteral obstruction. *J Endourol.* 2016; 30(4): 465–468.

19 Yakoubi R, Lemdani M, Monga M, Villers A, Koenig P. Is there a role for alpha-blockers in ureteral stent related symptoms? A systematic review and meta-analysis. *J Urol.* 2011; 186(3): 928–934.

20 Ho CH, Chen SC, Chung SD, *et al.* Determining the appropriate length

of a double-pigtail ureteral stent by both stent configurations and related symptoms. *J Endourol.* 2008; 22(7): 1427–1431.

21 Giannarini G, Keeley FX Jr, Valent F, *et al.* Predictors of morbidity in patients with indwelling ureteric stents: results of a prospective study using the validated Ureteric Stent Symptoms Questionnaire. *BJU Int.* 2011; 107(4): 648–654.

22 Dellis AE, Keeley FX Jr, Manolas V, Skolarikos AA. Role of alpha-blockers in the treatment of stent-related symptoms: a prospective randomized control study. *Urology.* 2014; 83(1): 56–61.

23 El-Nahas AR, Tharwat M, Elsaadany M, Mosbah A, Gaballah MA. A randomized controlled trial comparing alpha blocker (tamsulosin) and anticholinergic (solifenacin) in treatment of ureteral stent-related symptoms. *World J Urol.* 2016; 34(7): 963–968.

24 Kwon JK, Cho KS, Oh CK, *et al.* The beneficial effect of alpha-blockers for ureteral stent-related discomfort: systematic review and network meta-analysis

for alfuzosin versus tamsulosin versus placebo. *BMC Urol.* 2015; 15: 55.

25 Kawahara T, Ito H, Terao H, Yoshida M, Matsuzaki J. Ureteral stent encrustation, incrustation, and coloring: morbidity related to indwelling times. *J Endourol.* 2012; 26(2): 178–182.

26 Fam XI, Singam P, Ho CC, *et al.* Ureteral stricture formation after ureteroscope treatment of impacted calculi: a prospective study. *Korean J Urol.* 2015; 56(1): 63–67.

27 Tyritzis SI, Wiklund NP. Ureteral strictures revisited… trying to see the light at the end of the tunnel: a comprehensive review. *J Endourol.* 2015; 29(2): 124–136.

28 Duffy TP. Clinical problem-solving: an anatomy lesson. *N Engl J Med.* 1994; 331(5): 318–320.

29 Scheel PJ Jr, Feeley N. Retroperitoneal fibrosis: the clinical, laboratory, and radiographic presentation. *Medicine (Baltimore).* 2009; 88(4): 202–207.

30 Woodhouse CRJ. *Adolescent Urology and Long-Term Outcomes.* Oxford: Wiley, 2015.

6

Urinary Diversion

Christopher Woodhouse and Alex Kirkham

Introduction

From middle of the nineteenth century, when intra-abdominal surgery first became possible, urinary diversion was almost always by uretero-sigmoidostomy. The long-term results were poor, largely because of uncontrolled infections and metabolic complications. In the 1940s, Alexander Brunschwig, an American gynaecologist at Memorial Sloane Kettering, pioneered the procedure of total pelvic exenteration for locally advanced carcinoma of the cervix, which required a diversion other than via the rectum. The ileal conduit was devised by Eugene Bricker and reported in 1950 [1]. A Mr Rutzen of Chicago is credited by Bricker with designing the necessary appliance.

The results of ileal conduit after cystectomy were said to better than those after uretero-sigmoidostomy. However, it was more commonly used for children with congenital anomalies such as exstrophy and spina bifida. It is difficult, now, to appreciate the dramatic improvements that a conduit made to their lives. For example, 83% of 62 children undergoing ileal conduit for progressive renal deterioration were improved or stabilised according to the first postoperative intravenous urogram (IVU) [2]. In children who were diverted with normal kidneys, 70% were still normal after 10–16 years' follow-up [3].

The Procedures

Sixty-five years later, the ileal conduit remains the most common procedure for patients undergoing a cystectomy, although it is now seldom performed for paediatric patients. The design remains virtually the same as that originally described by Bricker. The features that have an impact on the postoperative imaging are as follows:

1 The alternative uretero-ileal anastomosis technique described by Wallace [4]. Theoretically, with the Wallace anastomosis, if there is an early leak both ureteric anastomoses may be lost. In an unrandomised comparison of 186 patients, the stricture rate with a Bricker was 3.7% and zero with a Wallace procedure [5]. In practice, the outcomes are much the same.
2 The length of ileum should be of sufficient length to reach without tension from the right iliac fossa to the abdominal wall, but no longer. In the very obese patient it may be difficult, or sometimes impossible, to pass the conduit through the abdominal wall without compromising the blood supply. It may be possible to overcome this problem using the modification of the stoma described by Turnbull (Figure 6.1) [6].
3 Isolated colon with an anti-reflux ureteric anastomosis has been used to make a urinary conduit. In practice, in only about 50% of cases is reflux prevented. There

Radiology and Follow-up of Urologic Surgery, First Edition. Edited by Christopher Woodhouse and Alex Kirkham.
© 2018 John Wiley & Sons Ltd. Published 2018 by John Wiley & Sons Ltd.

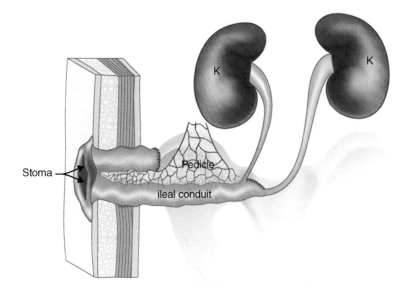

Figure 6.1 Diagram of the Turnbull stoma. Note that the stoma has a double blood supply as the pedicle supplies the two arms. On the surface it is usual for only a single orifice to be visible; for imaging, it must be recognised that there are two arms, one of which (usually the upper one) is blind ending.

has been a trend for it to reduce the incidence of renal scarring in children [7]. In adults, it has been claimed from a non-randomised and poorly matched series that there were fewer complications with a colon conduit after cystectomy; in children with follow-up to a maximum of 21 years, complication rates were similar [8, 9].

4 In patients having a total pelvic exenteration for cancer, particularly after radiotherapy, it is necessary to have a stoma each for urine and stool. Apart from the burden of two stomas, the further problem is that a vascularised abdominal flap is usually required to close the perineum which makes the positioning of one of the stomas difficult. It is possible to put both the stomas at the same site using descending colon, creating the double-barrelled stoma originally described by Carter *et al.* (Figure 6.2) [10]. With appropriate appliances, we have found no management problems. In 15 cases there have been fewer infections and parastomal hernias compared with seven similar patients who had bilateral stomas.

Clinical Follow-up of Ileal Conduits

The initial results of the ileal conduit were so good, in terms of improved kidneys, reduced infections and better cleanliness than a uretero-sigmoidostomy that many patients did not have any follow-up. It was not until 10–15 years after its first introduction that problems emerged [3, 11–13].

Postoperative Imaging

The 'Loopogram'

The most direct way of imaging the conduit is by instillation of contrast medium via the stoma. The aims of the study are to opacify the loop and demonstrate reflux into both ureters, opacifying both collecting systems and obtaining views to demonstrate intraluminal 'filling defects' suggesting epithelial pathology. The study is usually performed with a 10–14 Fr catheter and a balloon inflated in the intra-abdominal part of the loop (as close to the uretero-ileal anastomosis as possible, to reduce the effects of peristalsis on the efficacy of retrograde installation). The residual in the loop is measured on catheterisation, and between 30 and

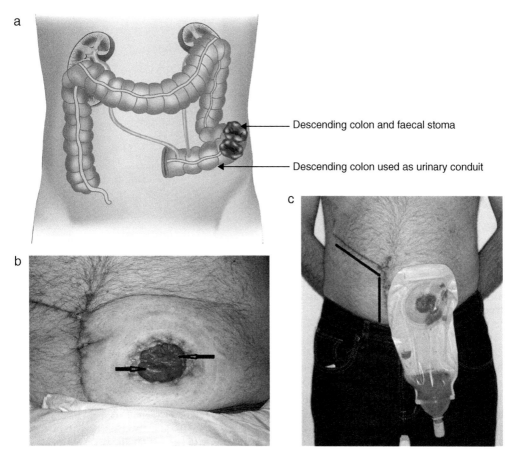

a

Descending colon and faecal stoma

Descending colon used as urinary conduit

b

c

Figure 6.2 (a) Diagram of the Carter double-barrelled stoma system. (b) The abdominal appearance of the Carter stoma with the orifices arrowed. (c) Following radiotherapy and total pelvic exenteration for locally advanced carcinoma of the rectum, the patient has a Carter stoma, showing the type of bag suitable for the drainage of faecal/urinary slurry; note the large drainage spout. A musculo-cutaneous flap based on the inferior epigastric vessels has been harvested approximately from the area outlined in black and used to close the perineum. The abdominal defect has been closed with a mesh which would make the formation of a right-sided stoma difficult.

150 mL of contrast instilled (some leakage is common via the stoma and indeed probably protects from overly high pressures during the study). The kidneys, ureters and bladder in two planes and images of the superficial loop are taken with a lateral view at 5 and 30 minutes after the procedure to assess emptying of the loop and upper tracts.

Loopograms may be carried out when there is a history of recurrent symptomatic urinary infection, or to look for reflux into the kidneys which would confirm *absence*

of upper tract obstruction (Figures 6.3 and 6.4).

It is occasionally indicated for the investigation of haematuria. However, although there are few specific data in this group of patients, CT urography is probably the more accurate method of investigation. It has superseded IVU and retrograde studies in the great majority of cases. Microscopic haematuria is almost always found in conduit urine and is seldom a sign of significant disease on its own. Gross haematuria requires

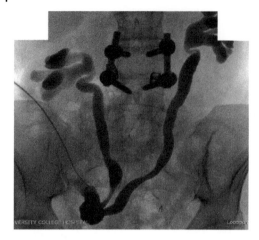

Figure 6.3 A single image from a loopogram study in a 55-year-old woman. The catheter is positioned in the middle of the loop, and the balloon inflated with 4 mL air. Reflux is seen to both kidneys, and both pelvi-caliceal systems are well shown.

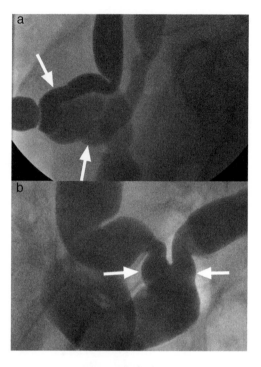

Figure 6.4 Two types of ureteric anastomosis. (a) The ureters enter the ileal loop in two discrete locations (Bricker type). (b) The ureters are joined into a short common ureteric segment before anastomosis to the loop (Wallace). Note the focus of narrowing in the loop in (a). This persisted on all views of the loop and was found to be a tumour at looposcopy; it was subsequently resected and the loop refashioned.

investigation as it would from a natural urinary tract. The most common causes are upper tract malignancy and stones. Some loops are too long and cause frequent symptomatic infections. Primary neoplasia of an ileal conduit is rare (Figures 6.5–6.8 and 6.9) [14].

The villous pattern of ileum is initially maintained after conduit formation. With time, there is villous atrophy which progresses at different rates among patients and within individual conduits. At 5 years' post conduit formation there will be some normal villi and some areas of atrophy. By a mean of 13 years, there is almost complete villous atrophy (Figure 6.10) [15].

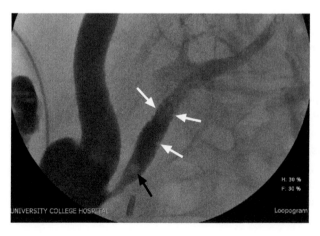

Figure 6.5 Multiple filling defects in the left ureter on a loopogram. Although the anastomosis appears moderately narrow, there was free reflux into the left ureter and the function of the left kidney was stable, indicating that it was not significantly obstructed. A single constant filling defect (arrows) might raise the possibility of a ureteric tumour, but the multiple small filling defects (constant compared with a year ago) suggested ureteritis cystica. This was confirmed at ureteroscopy.

Figure 6.6 Methods for imaging a ureteric tumour. Ultrasound (US) initially showed increasing hydronephrosis in the right kidney. (a) A loopogram showed reflux into only a small distal part of the right ureter, with an irregular upper margin suggesting tumour (white arrow; a black arrow indicates the contralateral ureter). (b) A right nephrostomy was placed, and shows a nephrostogram showing the upper limit of the tumour (arrow). (c) Only the CT scan fully demonstrates the length and size of the ureteric tumour (arrows).

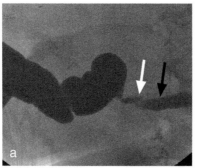

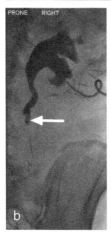

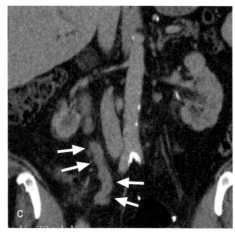

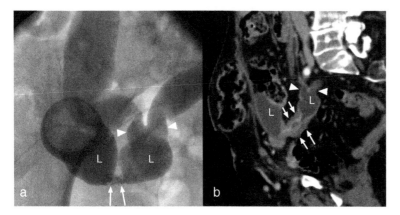

Figure 6.7 Stricture of an ileal conduit on loopogram and CT. The stricture (constant on multiple images) is well shown on the loopogram (a, arrows) but it is impossible to determine the wall thickness. Ureters (arrow heads) are dilated. (b) An oblique sagittally reconstructed enhanced CT image (60 s after IV contrast). The smoothly, moderately thickened ileal wall is demonstrated (arrows). In both images L = loop. The imaging appearances would go with malignancy, but biopsy showed only chronic active inflammation.

Ultrasound

The most serious complication of the ileal conduit is obstructive renal failure. This is best identified initially by ultrasound (US). Some dilatation of the upper tracts is common in patients with ileal conduits and may not be associated with obstruction or significant functional deterioration.

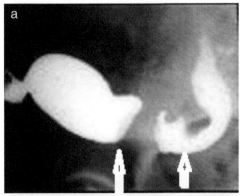

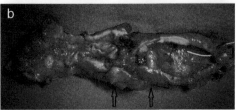

Figure 6.8 (a) Combined loopogram and antegrade nephrostogram showing complete obstruction of the conduit with an irregular mass (between the arrows). (b) Fresh surgical specimen from the same patient showing the tumour between the arrows. There are stents in the ureters. Histology showed an adenocarcinoma.

loopogram or MAG3 isotope renogram. MAG3 is the standard investigation for obstruction; however, if a loopogram shows reflux, obstruction is unlikely and other information may be gathered from visualisation of the whole renal drainage system. Obstruction may be at the lower end of the ureter, the anastomosis to the conduit or at stomal level. US may in some cases identify a distended loop (Figure 6.11), although this finding is operator dependent, and distension does not necessarily imply obstruction.

Stomal obstruction may be seen on abdominal examination, confirmed, if possible, by the insertion of a small catheter to drain the residual urine (Figure 6.12). Obstruction by a stricture of the conduit itself is rare, and should raise the possibility of tumour (Figure 6.7 and 6.8.).

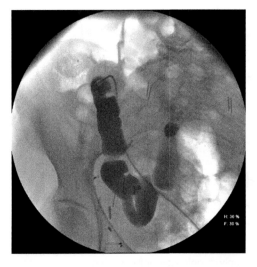

Figure 6.9 Loopogram showing an unnecessarily long conduit looping down into the pelvis.

Progressive dilatation, particularly when associated with a rising serum creatinine level, requires further investigation by

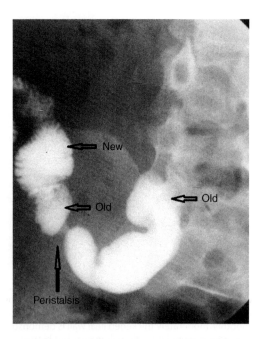

Figure 6.10 Loopogram of an ileal conduit. The old section, which was formed in early childhood, shows smooth walls with no villi. In adulthood, after two pregnancies and with increasing obesity, it had become too short and a new segment was added on to lengthen it about a year before this X-ray. The new segment shows normal villi and haustral folds.

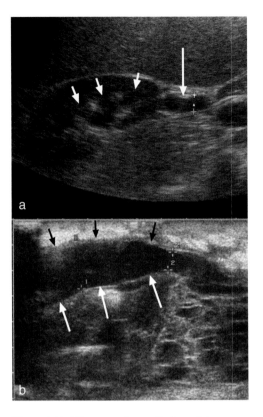

Figure 6.11 US 5 years after an ileal conduit showing: (a) mild dilatation of the collecting system in the kidney (short arrows), and upper ureter (long arrow). (b) a moderately distended loop with no evidence of a focal lesion (between arrows).

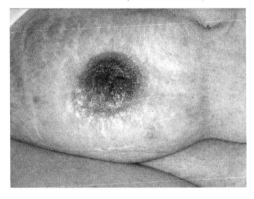

Figure 6.12 Clinical photograph showing a stenosed ileal stoma causing obstruction of the conduit

Nephrostomy and Antegrade Imaging

Although it is sometimes possible to insert a ureteric stent endoscopically through the conduit, in the presence of an anastomotic stricture it is most often impossible. An antegrade nephrostomy is usually the first line procedure and allows a definitive diagnosis. It may be combined with dilatation and stenting of the most common cause – a benign stricture (Figure 6.13).

Stenting allows the kidney to recover as much as is possible and gains time while working out what to do next. Unfortunately, the function of the obstructed kidney may be so poor that it is not worth saving.

In the long term, balloon dilatation has a poor outcome, with up to 85% re-strictured at 1 year and up to 95% by 3 years [16]. Longer term success usually requires a permanent JJ stent which is changed every 3 months [17]. Metal stents are reported to fall out in 90% of cases by a mean of 21 days [18].

The best outcomes with balloon dilatation are associated with strictures of <1 cm occurring more than 6 months postoperatively, not following abdominal radiotherapy and from kidneys with more than 35% of total function on isotope scanning [16].

Nonetheless, an aggressive policy to identify and manage obstruction is essential. Renal failure can occur in more than 16% of patients after ileal conduit diversion, often through neglect of follow-up. New cases are found as late as 5 years postoperatively. Kidneys that are abnormal pre-operatively are at greater risk [19]. Open repair has about a 90% success rate at 1 year but then there is a progressive rate of recurrence, at least up to 4 years, by which time about 25% will have re-stenosed [16, 20].

Monitoring of Asymptomatic Patients

The incidence of renal obstruction, which is usually symptomless, mandates regular supervision on its own. There is no high level evidence to guide its protocol.

As most surgeons will protect the ureteric anastomosis with stents for a period postoperatively, it is sensible to perform a renal

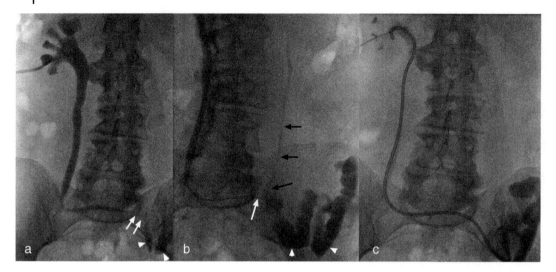

Figure 6.13 Stenting of an anastomotic stricture. (a) An initial nephrostogram shows only a small amount of drainage past an anastomotic stricture (arrows) into the conduit (arrowheads). A MAG3 study had shown impaired function and delayed drainage. (b) The stricture has been crossed with a wire, and there is now reflux from the Wallace anastomosis into the contralateral ureter (black arrows). (c) A JJ stent has been placed and the kidney is draining well into the loop (note the empty collecting system).

ultrasound and measure the serum creatinine within a few days of stent removal to establish a baseline and to detect an early disaster. Thereafter there are no guidelines, let alone any that are validated for the monitoring of an ileal conduit in the asymptomatic patient. Annual review has become customary. This fits in with our experience of ileal conduit patients with a variety of benign and malignant underlying diagnoses [21]. We are only aware of one patient who went from a normal state to end-stage renal failure in less than a year. Ultrasound at end stage showed bilateral shrunken kidneys and the patient probably had unrecognised renal disease rather than obstruction. Another patient developed bilateral obstruction, sequentially at about 4 and 6 months after the previous stable ultrasound at 3 years' post conduit formation (unpublished data). Aside from these, the development of obstruction has been a slow process.

A protocol for monitoring of the conduit is shown in Table 6.1. The underlying diagnosis for which the conduit was needed, most often cancer, may require its own, more intensive, monitoring.

Although the very serious complication of vitamin B_{12} deficiency can be found after ileal conduit formation, it is rare. It should not occur until at least 4 years after conduit formation when the body store would be exhausted *if there was absolutely no further absorption*. No cases are recorded in the detailed follow-up of 412 patients up to nearly 30 years in the series of Madersbacher *et al.* [22] (although it may not have been routinely measured).

Management of Bacteriuria and Sepsis

In clinical practice, there is great difficulty in managing alleged urinary tract infections (UTI) in patients with conduits. This is partly because many patients and general practitioners ascribe almost any symptom, especially if accompanied by 'smelly urine', to UTI and partly because most patients do have bacteriuria for much of the time but fail to appreciate that it is actually symptomless.

The problem lies in renal infection. There is no difficulty in making a diagnosis of

Table 6.1 Suggested protocol for the follow-up of asymptomatic patients with an ileal conduit.

Procedure	Frequency	Year 1		Year 2 onwards	Year 5 onwards
		3 months	6 months	Annually	Annually
Inspect stoma	Every visit				
Blood pressure	Every visit				
Urine protein (stix)	Every visit				
Full blood count	Every visit				
Serum creatinine	Every visit				
Serum B_{12}					Every visit[a]
Urinary tract ultrasound		Yes	Yes	Yes	Yes[b]

a) Vitamin B_{12} deficiency with a standard length ileal conduit and without previous abdominal radiotherapy is rare and routine measurement is not undertaken in many units.
b) Annual renal ultrasound after 6 years in asymptomatic patients with previously normal kidneys has low pick-up rate; if the other parameters remain normal, biennial examination may be acceptable.

acute pyelonephritis in a diverted patient because it is exactly the same as in anyone else. There is high fever, often with rigors and pain, and tenderness in the affected kidney. Bilateral synchronous pyelonephritis is rare. On investigation, the white blood count and C-reactive protein (CRP) levels are raised. There is increasing use of more sophisticated biomarkers of infection such as procalcitonin or preseptin both for diagnosis and prognostication [23]. Ultrasound may show an oedematous kidney. Hydronephrosis will raise the possibility of a pyonephrosis.

The critical issue is that, for a urinary tract infection to require antibiotics, it must be making the patient 'ill' in some way. There may be malaise, low grade fever and other symptoms that are recognizable to individual patients.

With a suspicious group of symptoms, a catheter specimen of urine should be sent for culture. Urine from the 'ostomy' bag will always contain bacteria. Ideally, a catheter should be passed as deeply as possible into the conduit and a further catheter passed through it to obtain an uncontaminated specimen. The residual urine in a conduit should ideally be <15 mL but many patients have much larger residuals apparently without any problems. A higher residual may indicate an excessively long and poorly draining conduit (Figure 6.9) [24].

'Clean catch' urine from the stoma may be acceptable and if it is sterile will out rule an infection. A positive culture may not prove that a significant infection is present and further evidence from inflammatory markers is needed [25].

It is not surprising that UTI is greatly over-diagnosed. As with all other complications, the longer the follow-up, the higher the incidence becomes. With strict attention to diagnostic criteria, an incidence as low as 3% after a mean of 11 years has been reported [26]. Others give 8–11% at 5 years, which seems more probable.

References

1 Bricker EM. Bladder substitution after pelvic exenteration. *Urol Clin North Am.* 1950; 30: 1511–1521.

2 Stevens PS, Eckstein HB. Ileal conduit urinary diversion in children. *Br J Urol.* 1971; 51: 466–470.

3 Shapiro SR, Lebovitz R, Colodny AH. The fate of 90 children with an ileal conduit urinary diversion 10 years later. *J Urol.* 1975; 114: 289–295.

4 Wallace DM. Uretero-ileostomy. *Br J Urol.* 1970; 42: 529–534.

5 Kouba E, Sands M, Lentz A, Wallen E, Pruthi RS. A comparison of the Bricker versus Wallace ureteroileal anastomosis in patients undergoing urinary diversion for bladder cancer. *J Urol.* 2007; 178(3 Pt 1): 945–948.

6 Bloom DA, Lieskovsky G, Rainwater G, Skinner DG. The Turnbull loop stoma. *J Urol.* 1983; 129(4): 715–718.

7 Hill JT, Ransley PG. The colonic conduit: a better method of urinary diversion? *Br J Urol.* 1985; 55: 629–631.

8 Pycha A, Comploj E, Martini T, *et al.* Comparison of complications in three incontinent urinary diversions. *Eur Urol.* 2008; 54(4): 825–832.

9 Elder DD, Moisey CU, Rees RWM. A long-term follow up of the colonic conduit operation in children. *Br J Urol.* 1979; 51: 462–465.

10 Carter MF, Dalton DP, Garnett JE. The double-barreled wet colostomy: long term experience with the first 11 patients. *J Urol.* 1994; 156: 2312–2315.

11 Dunn M, Roberts JBM, Smith PJB, Slade N. The long term results of ileal conduit diversion in children. *Br J Urol.* 1979; 51: 458–461.

12 Jones MA, Breckman B, Hendry WF. Life with an ileal conduit: results of questionaire surveys of patients and urological surgeons. *Br J Urol.* 1980; 52: 21–25.

13 Neal DE. Complications of ileal conduit diversion in adults with cancer followed up for at least five years. *Br Med J (Clin Res Ed).* 1985; 290(6483): 1695–1697.

14 Austen M, Kalble T. Secondary malignancies in different forms of urinary diversion using isolated gut. *J Urol.* 2004; 172: 831–838.

15 Deane AM, Woodhouse CRJ, Parkinson MC. Histological changes in ileal conduits. *J Urol.* 1984; 132: 1108–1111.

16 DiMarco DS, LeRoy AJ, Thieling S, Bergstralh EJ, Segura JW. Long-term results of treatment for ureteroenteric strictures. *Urology.* 2001; 58(6): 909–913.

17 Pappas P, Stravodimos KG, Kapetanakis T, *et al.* Ureterointestinal strictures following Bricker ileal conduit: management via a percutaneous approach. *Int Urol Nephrol.* 2008; 40(3): 621–627.

18 Garg T, Guralnick ML, Langenstroer P, *et al.* Resonance metallic ureteral stents do not successfully treat ureteroenteric strictures. *J Endourol.* 2009; 23(7): 1199–1201.

19 Gilbert SM, Lai J, Saigal CS, Gore JL. Downstream complications following urinary diversion. *J Urol.* 2013; 190(3): 916–922.

20 Nassar OA, Alsafa ME. Experience with ureteroenteric strictures after radical cystectomy and diversion: open surgical revision. *Urology.* 2011; 78(2): 459–465.

21 Bakke A, Jensen KM, Jonsson O, *et al.* The rationale behind recommendations for follow-up after urinary diversion: an evidence-based approach. *Scand J Urol Nephrol.* 2007; 41(4): 261–269.

22 Madersbacher S, Schmidt J, Eberle JM, *et al.* Long-term outcome of ileal conduit diversion. *J Urol.* 2003; 169(3): 985–990.

23 Liu B, Chen YX, Yin Q, Zhao YZ, Li CS. Diagnostic value and prognostic evaluation of Presepsin for sepsis in an emergency department. *Crit Care.* 2013; 17(5): R244.

24 Frank PP, Pernet M, Jonas U. Ileal conduit diversion: early and late results of 132 cases in a 25 year period. *World J Urol.* 1985; 3: 140–144.

25 Mahoney M, Baxter K, Burgess J, *et al.* Procedure for obtaining a urine sample from a urostomy, ileal conduit, and colon conduit: a best practice guideline for clinicians. *J Wound Ostomy Continence Nurs.* 2013; 40(3): 277–279.

26 Lopez PP, Moreno Valle JA, Espinosa L, *et al.* Enterocystoplasty in children with neuropathic bladders: long-term follow-up. *J Pediatr Urol.* 2008; 4(1): 27–31.

7

Ureteric Reconstruction and Replacement

Christopher Woodhouse and Aslam Sohaib

Introduction

It is sad to have to record that the ureter is most often in need of repair because of damage by doctors. Surgeons may cut it; radiotherapists may burn it; radiologists may penetrate it during interventional procedures. Isolated trauma is uncommon but the ureter may be damaged as a part of a multi-organ injury of the abdomen [1]. Several diseases may obstruct the ureter, the most common of which in the Western world is cancer; in some countries tuberculosis and schistosomiasis are more common causes. Patients may damage their own ureters especially with ketamine which is a newly emerging drug of abuse (Figure 7.1) [2]. The cause of the ureteric damage is most influential in the selection of the type of repair.

The best tissue with which to repair the ureter is the ureter itself. If that is not feasible, tubularised bladder is the next choice. Autologous tissue foreign to the urinary tract is the least satisfactory. Synthetic stents and nephrostomy tubes are very useful in the short term. Reconstruction and replacement of the ureter is an exercise in imaginative use of the available techniques.

Procedures

Stents and Nephrostomies

An obstructed ureter will cause irreversible deterioration in renal function at least as early as 2 months from onset [3]. Ureteric stents will usually, but not always, establish adequate downward drainage and allow recovery of renal function. A percutaneous nephrostomy can be more effective and sometimes is the only possible option. Either stents or a nephrostomy will sometimes dry up a ureteric fistula. They are generally regarded as short-term measures, but occasionally circumstances require them to be permanent.

Uretero-pyelostomy

Anastomosis of the upper ureter to the renal pelvis was originally described by Anderson and Hynes [4] for the management of an obstructing retrocaval ureter (Figure 7.2). A damaged upper ureter can be salvaged by the

Radiology and Follow-up of Urologic Surgery, First Edition. Edited by Christopher Woodhouse and Alex Kirkham.
© 2018 John Wiley & Sons Ltd. Published 2018 by John Wiley & Sons Ltd.

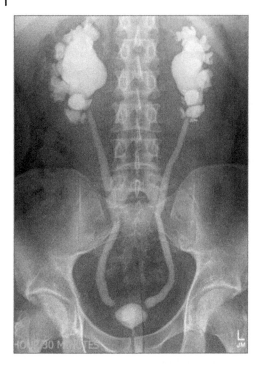

Figure 7.1 Standard intravenous urogram (IVU) of a patient with urinary tract damage from ketamine abuse. There is bilateral hydronephrosis. The ureters are drawn medially and rigid in appearance. The apparent obstruction at the lower ends is in the intra-mural portion (cystogram showed no obstruction). The bladder is small and thick walled. *Source:* Woodhouse 2015 [52]. Reproduced with permission of John Wiley and Sons.

same technique. The more dilated the renal pelvis, the longer the length of damaged ureter that can be repaired.

Uretero-calycostomy

If the kidney is chronically dilated and the lower pole calyx close to the surface, the ureter can be anastomosed to it. However, there are few occasions on which it is feasible.

Trans-uretero-ureterostomy

Much the most useful technique for repair of the mid ureter is to pass the surviving upper ureter across the retroperitoneum and anastomose it to the contralateral ureter. There have been anecdotal concerns that either the donor or the recipient ureter (or

both) would be damaged. However, in a retrospective series of 253 cases, virtually no complications were encountered, but in particular no ureters became damaged as a result of the repair [5].

Both experimental and clinical experiences confirm that both ureters drain into a bladder or reservoir. The host ureter has the dominant function in that its electromyographic impulses continue to pass down to the distal (common) ureter while those of the donor ureter do not [6]. This does not prevent the drainage from the donor ureter or cause hydronephrosis.

Ureteric Re-implantation

For a damaged lower ureter, direct re-implantation into the bladder using a subepithelial tunnel is the procedure of choice. If the compromised lower ureter is only a centimetre or two, the bladder can be fixed to the psoas to prevent tension on the anastomosis. For longer sections of missing ureter it is necessary to raise a flap of bladder known as a Boari (Figure 7.3). The Boari flap is a most useful means of salvaging the ureter using urothelial lined tissue. Providing the bladder has not been damaged, particularly by irradiation, a long flap can be raised which will usually reach to the upper third of the ureter especially if a downward nephropexy is carried out as well [7]. It can sometimes reach as high as the renal pelvis, especially in females.

Apart from minor leaks in the perioperative period in about 3% of patients, long-term complications are rare. There is no difference in outcome among those having a simple re-implantation, a psoas hitch or a Boari flap [3]. The important technical point is to make a proper assessment of the ureteric defect and choose the operation which will provide a tension-free implantation with an adequate tunnel. If in doubt it is safest to perform a Boari flap.

The Boari flap is versatile and can be modified to drain both ureters, either by combining it with a trans-uretero-ureterostomy

Figure 7.2 Enhanced coronal CT image to show a retrocaval ureter. There is a stent in the ureter (arrowed) which can be seen curling behind the inferior vena cava. The kidney is dilated.

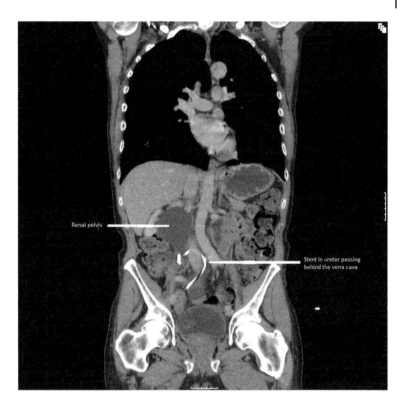

Renal pelvis

Stent in ureter passing behind the vena cava

a b c

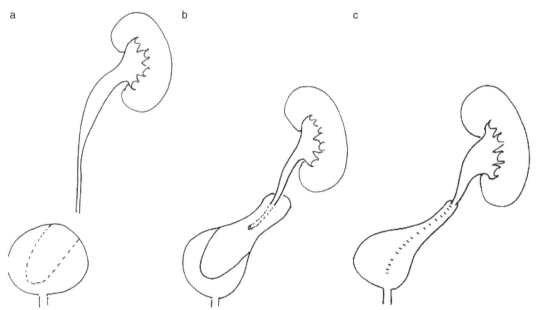

Figure 7.3 Formation of a Boari flap. (a) The flap has been marked out on the bladder; note the broad base and curved distal end. (b) The flap has been raised and the ureter tunnelled into the sub-epithelium. (c) The flap has been closed as a tube.

(TUU) or by bring one ureter across to the other side and implanting them separately into the top of the flap. It can also be used to repair the infective causes of ureteric stricture such as schistosomiasis and tuberculosis once appropriate chemotherapy has been completed and the extent of the stricture defined [8, 9]. In a small prospective controlled trial in patients with schistosomiasis of the ureters, Boari flap was found to be superior to a Girgis triangular flap or ileal interposition at a mean follow-up of 20 months [10].

All of these techniques can also be used in children [11].

Autotransplantation

Removal of a kidney and moving it down to the pelvis was originally championed for the management of low grade transitional cell carcinoma in the collecting system or ureter combined with bench surgery as an alternative to nephrectomy [12]. Indications have expanded with time, especially as the operation can be performed laparoscopically. There are several reports of its use for complex ureteric injuries and strictures. A short length of upper ureter can be implanted in the bladder or the renal pelvis can be anastomosed directly to it [13, 14].

Intestine

If it is impossible to find a way of reconstructing the ureter with urothelial-lined tissue, intestine can be used. The original descriptions were of a direct anastomosis of a length of ileum between the renal pelvis and the bladder (an ileal chute). The large dead space that this created predisposed to infection and the complications associated with storage of urine in intestinal segments. Nonetheless, it remains a very simple technique and most patients do well. The wide bore allows the passage of renal stones without colic. It was for recurrent stone formers that the chute was particularly popularised.

To reduce the amount of dead space and length of intestine needed, narrow tubes have been used. The use of the appendix is at the level of case reports. It is not normally long enough to replace a whole ureter and its lumen is often small, around 8 Fr. However, it has been used successfully in 9 of 10 children with a mean follow-up of 2.5 years (range 1–72 months). Interestingly, it was implanted in an anti-peristaltic direction; one child developed hydronephrosis [15]. It may be useful in association with a Boari flap. It has also been used after incising on its anti-mesenteric border to form a sheet with which to augment an opened ureteric stricture [16].

A tailored ureteric replacement can be formed from ileum or colon using the Yang–Monti technique. A single segment will not replace the whole ureter, but a double or spiral Yang–Monti can be made long enough, especially if colon is used with or without a Boari flap [17].

Complex Lower Urinary Tract Reconstruction

Damage to the ureter may be a part of extensive intra-abdominal and pelvic injury, usually from trauma, but occasionally from radiotherapy or surgery. The ureteric reconstruction then has to be part of a complex lower tract reconstruction. Any of the available techniques for ureteric replacement can be combined with any of the standard bladder replacements. An example is shown in Figure 7.4, but there are many variations in the literature as case reports or small series, including implanting a reconstructed ureter into the sigmoid colon.

Other Materials and Experimental Techniques

Several substitute materials have been tried experimentally and clinically. With a few honourable exceptions, negative outcomes are missing from the literature. There may well be a wide range materials that have been tried, found wanting and not reported. Some of the experiments have been carried out on ureteric defects that could be bridged quite

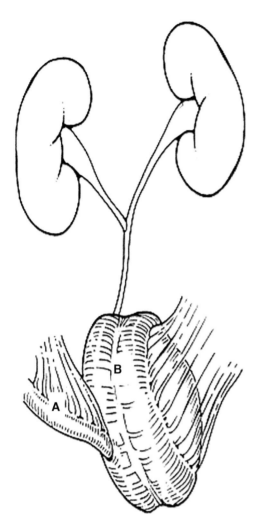

Figure 7.4 Complex lower urinary tract reconstruction following an extensive crush injury to the pelvis with loss of the bladder, prostate and lower right ureter. A right to left trans-uretero-ureterostomy (TUU) has been formed. The bladder has been replaced with an intestinal reservoir (B) which is drained by an appendiceal Mitrofanoff channel (A). The left ureter has been implanted into the reservoir.

easily with urothelial tissues using one of the techniques above. Others, although successful in animals, have not found their way into clinical practice. A further discouragement to experimentation in this field is that the need for non-urothelial tissues is small.

The most widely used tissue is small intestinal submucosa (SIS) which is used as a scaffold on which urothelial cells may grow or be grafted after tissue culture. When used as a patch on a partially excised segment of pig ureter, urothelium grows in well and the ureter functions normally [18]. When used as a tube, even with a stent, the in-growth of urothelium is patchy and the tube obliterates [19]. The use of cultured urothelium is no better, except when a de-mucosalised Yang–Monti vascularised tube is used as the scaffold [20]. Recently, urothelial cells from human adipose-derived stem cells have been more reliable in forming sheets of urothelium [21].

A tube of buccal mucosa has been used in five patients to replace a strictured ureter. The defect was between 3.5 and 5 cm and resulted from non-malignant causes. The longest follow-up was 39 months (mean 24 months) and all patients remained unobstructed [22]. Vein grafts have been used in a rat model. A good ureter resulted providing a stent was used until healing was complete [23].

Clinical Follow-up and Complications

Stents and Nephrostomies

Plastic tubes of various types are most often used for temporary protection of the kidneys pending a definitive intervention or for a short time thereafter. Longer term use is usually for malignant obstruction in patients with a poor prognosis. The typical survival after stenting in this group is shown in Figure 7.5. The short survival may influence the choice of stent, timing of their renewal and, indeed, whether a stent should be inserted at all.

A very wide range of immediate complications has been reported including the stent being too long or too short; being impossible to pass; being passed out of the ureter; and becoming knotted. It is to be hoped that these complications are quickly recognised and corrected endoscopically.

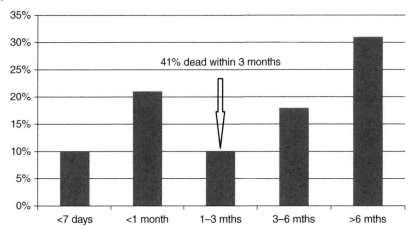

Figure 7.5 Chart to show the survival of patients after palliative ureteric stenting in malignant disease (audit data 2012 Royal Marsden Hospital, London). *Source:* Woodhouse 2010 [53]. Reproduced with permission of Elsevier.

Temporary stents should be removed as soon as they are no longer needed. There is no good evidence to guide the timing of exchange of stents that are required for long periods or even permanently. In view of the speed with which encrustation can occur, scheduled exchanges at 1 year seems ambitious especially as medical schedules have a habit of slipping for administrative or clinical reasons. Six-monthly exchange is a good target and should allow for some slippage. Even with this schedule, occasional patients are going to develop significant encrustation before their next appointment. With those who have to have lifelong stents, it may be possible to define the length of time it takes to form encrustation in that patient and arrange a schedule accordingly.

Much the most important part of internal stent follow-up is to ensure that it is removed or changed in a timely manner. A check should be made that it has not broken with the upper end left behind (Figure 7.6). No stent devised to date has been shown to be immune to encrustation; some are said to be better than others but only based on in vitro experiments which do not mimic the natural environment of the urinary tract. In clinical practice, sufficient encrustation to make removal of a stent difficult has been found after 2 months. In that report the mean time to developing clinically significant encrustation was 11.4 months (range 2–39 months).

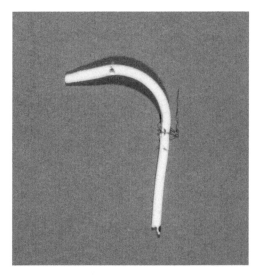

Figure 7.6 Broken upper end of a ureteric stent. It had been put in at open surgery and the presence of a holding stitch had not been recorded and it broke on attempted removal.

The most extensive encrustation in which the whole stent is embedded in stone (grade V on the scale of Acosta-Miranda *et al.*) occurs in forgotten stents after 2 years or so. Progressively more complex endoscopic or percutaneous procedures are needed for stent extraction with more extensive encrustation. Acosta-Miranda *et al.* [24] have described a useful algorithm. Faster encrustation is associated with infection, a history of recurrent stone formation and dehydration.

Stents are colonised with bacteria or fungi in up to 97% of cases [25]. Efforts to manufacture stents that resist colonisation have not been successful [26]. Different organisms may colonise different parts of the stent and may be different from those cultured from urine. The longer the stent is in situ the greater is the incidence of positive urine culture reaching nearly 50% after 90 days of dwell time [27]. Although bacteria predispose to encrustation, a positive urine culture should only be treated if there are symptoms. Prophylaxis is likely to lead to the development of resistant organisms [28]. The incidence of symptomatic urinary infection is difficult to determine as many patients are given antibiotics in the community for irritable bladder symptoms probably unrelated to bacteriuria. Systemic infection has been reported in 3.6% of adults and 10% of children. In the children's series, the indication for stenting was pyeloplasty which may itself have caused infection. The organisms cultured from blood or urine were not always the same as those found on the stents [29, 30].

It has been claimed that 80% of patients with indwelling stents have pain that affects their daily living, mostly in the urinary tract, but also affecting sexuality (32%) and preventing full-time work (58%). Although this study was meticulously performed, the indications for stenting are not given which makes it impossible to know whether patients requiring long-term stenting are so affected [31]. The clinical impression is that patients with long-term stents, especially those who have had chronic obstruction, have few if any symptoms. Bladder symptoms can be caused by stent migration or a lower coil that crosses the midline. They can be reduced with the use of stents with at least the lower coil made of a soft material [32]. Ureteric and, to a lesser extent bladder, pain can be reduced with alpha-blocking drugs [33]. The addition of anticholinergics does not help [34].

A clinical problem that has been the subject of little research is the failure of a stent to drain, manifested by declining renal function. It is a phenomenon that can occur at any time after insertion. It has been found that, at least in a pig model, stents inhibit peristalsis but this does not act as a complete obstruction; it does cause minor hydronephrosis [35]. The most obvious cause is that the stent is blocked or crushed by an obstructing tumour. These possibilities can only be checked by passing a guide wire up the stent via a cystoscope or inserting a nephrostomy. It is occasionally found that a stent, although not obstructed, will not drain a kidney while a nephrostomy will do so. This may be because the column of urine in the drainage tube of a nephrostomy exerts a negative pressure while a chronically dilated renal pelvis is unable to generate enough pressure to push the urine down a stent [36]. In some patients, metal stents or two standard stents in tandem may resolve the problem [37]. The failure rate with the former is at least 28% and there are no firm data on the latter in this context [38].

There is a variety of metallic stents available which are more expensive but last longer. There are few long-term results. Two series of 10 and 11 years of experience but with only a mean follow-up 15 and 16 months, respectively, suggest that up to 25% have to be replaced. Expanding stents have been associated with fistulation from the ureter into bowel, vagina and major arteries in patients who have had radiation and/or major pelvic surgery [39]. Although many of the replacements were for symptomatic problems, urine culture and measurement of serum creatinine are necessary every 3 months. Plain X-ray to detect encrustation or migration are needed twice a year [40, 41].

Long-term percutaneous nephrostomies are difficult to manage. The dressing over the puncture site has to be changed about every 2 weeks by a clinician who understands the technique and can be trusted not to pull the tube out. The tube should be changed every 6 weeks, but in practice deterioration of the tube and accidental removal are common reasons for putting in a new one.

Reconstruction with Urothelium

The reconstructions using anastomosis of ureter to renal pelvis, ureter to ureter and ureteric re-implantation with or without a Boari flap are remarkably successful. Their follow-up and long-term outcomes are almost identical. Late stricture is rare unless there is progression of the underlying problem, especially radiotherapy, schistosomiasis or tuberculosis.

The function and appearance of the kidneys after obstruction has been most studied in patients after repair of pelvi-ureteric obstruction. It seems likely that repair of a damaged upper ureter by essentially the same techniques, will have the same outcomes (see Chapter 4). The appearances on standard imaging do not usually return to normal but are improved in up to 90% and stable on follow-up at least to 5 years [42]. However, the outflow returns to a non-obstructed pattern but with sluggish transit (Figure 7.7).

The clinical follow-up after TUU is similar. There is no significant change in the estimated glomerular filtration rate (eGFR), although the means for whole series do show marginal improvements such as 81–83 mL/min. Pre-existing hydronephrosis may improve. The most important investigation is a renogram to confirm absence of obstruction. As with the situation after pelvi-ureteric junction obstruction reconstruction, flow is sluggish but obstruction eliminated (Figure 7.8). Late obstruction is almost always caused by progression of malignancy. Occasionally, hydronephrosis is caused by 'yo-yo' reflux of urine from one kidney to other, unassociated with obstruction or loss of function [43].

In children in whom TUU is most often performed as a part of a complex reconstruction for congenital anomalies, normal calibre ureters remain normal and dilated ones improve or even return to normal in three-quarters of cases [44].

Progressive renal failure is only seen in patients with impaired renal function before surgery. A relief of obstruction may delay the

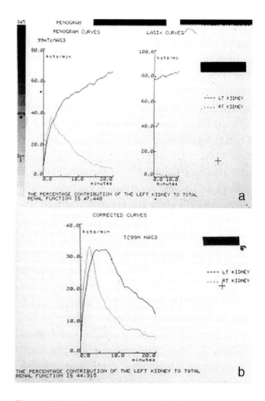

Figure 7.7 MAG3 renograms (a) before and (b) 1 year after left pelvi-ureteric junction repair. Note that the contribution of the left kidney to overall function has not changed significantly. being 47% before surgery and 44% afterwards. The left kidney curve shows classic obstruction before surgery and sluggish transit but unobstructed pattern afterwards.

onset of end-stage renal failure but does not prevent it occurring eventually.

The same outcomes are found for re-implantation into the bladder either with a psoas hitch or with a Boari flap. The flap looks remarkably like a rather irregular ureter (Figure 7.9), although short ones look broader, similar to a rabbit's ear (see Figure 8.9). About 80% of ureters and kidneys normalise or improve in appearance. Renal function outcomes are reported to be less good than with anastomosis higher up the ureter. Even in patients with normal renal function pre-operatively, deterioration may be found in up to 6% of patients, mostly men over 60 years old [3]. This finding is probably a result of case selection in a group of patients with complex diagnoses. The

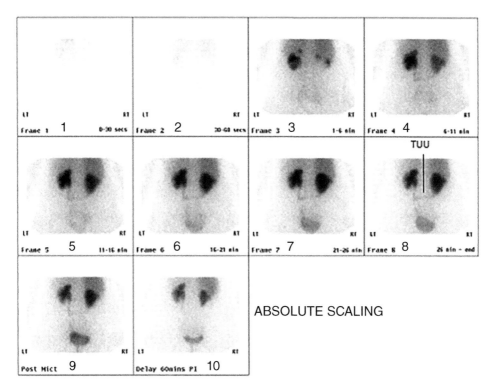

Figure 7.8 MAG3 study after a right to left TUU (marked with a line in frame 8). Note that both kidneys are dilated and there is sluggish flow. Delayed picture at 1 hour (frame 10) shows good but incomplete clearance. There is no obstruction and the renal function remained normal.

deterioration was not defined and seems not to be clinically significant. Long-term results in patients with the relatively simple lower ureteric injuries at surgery are lacking but late stricture of the anastomosis is seldom reported [45]. However, in the series of Noble *et al.* [5] six of 253 developed strictures of the distal host ureter because of progression of the original disease.

For all of these repairs, therefore, follow-up is only required for any underlying progressive disease. If renal function is at or near normal and renogram shows no obstruction at 1 year, no further follow-up is needed for the ureteric reconstruction itself.

Autotransplantation

The most high risk of the options is autotransplantaion. In the series of 305 transplants reported by Flatmark *et al.* [46], there was a 4% 90-day mortality. This high figure reflects the extensive co-morbidities of many of the patients who were often elderly and atherosclerotic [46]. Figures from two very experienced transplant centres give a graft loss rate of 3.6% and 8.7%, respectively, the latter figure being from a series exclusively of patients with ureteric damage [46, 47]. Other series report complication rates of Clavien III or above of 10–15% and occasional early graft failures [14, 48, 49].

The clinical follow-up for the surgical aspects of renal transplantation are covered in Chapter 2. With autotransplantaion there is no immunosuppression. The follow-up, therefore, is for renal function. Most series report on autotransplantation for all causes together and those for ureteric replacement alone are few.

For all diagnoses, good data on the outcome of the autotransplanted kidney come from a series of 69 patients (of 305) who had

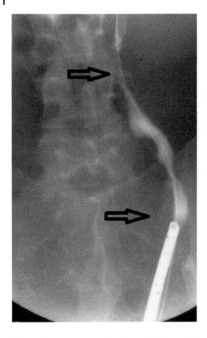

Figure 7.9 Retrograde X-ray of a Boari flap. It extends between the arrows. A guide wire is in place in the flap and ureter. Note that the lumen of the flap is larger than that of a normal ureter but not as large as the cystoscope (20 Fr). The lumen is somewhat irregular but there are no diverticula (see also Figure 8.9).

only one functioning kidney. At follow-up from 6 to 108 months, 76% had stable renal function [46]. From another series of 52 patients, four (8%) whose autograft survived the operation subsequently failed between 15 and 48 months [13]. As late failure can occur, monitoring should continue for life.

Intestine

As with the other methods of ureteric replacement, ileum seems to work well with good long-term outcomes. On imaging, it looks much the same as an ileal conduit (Figure 7.10). Imaging at 6 months to define anatomy can be by cystogram, magnetic resonance imaging (MRI) urogram or computed tomography (CT) urogram (Figure 7.11). There is a tendency to make ileal ureters too long which increases the incidence of infection and may even cause

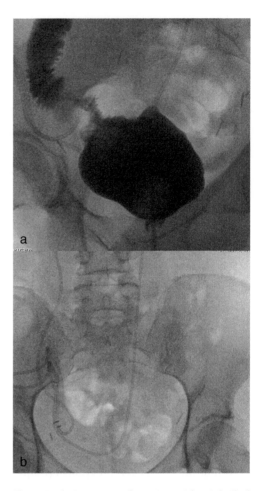

Figure 7.10 Cystogram of a patient with a right ileal ureter (a) during filling and (b) after bladder emptying. Ureteric stents are still in place as these are taken early after surgery to confirm healing in a heavily irradiated pelvis. During filling there is free reflux into the ileal ureter but complete drainage after bladder emptying.

obstruction by kinking. However, in some patients an excessively long ileal ureter causes no problems (Figure 7.12).

Anastomotic stricture is rare, especially after the first year. Renal function is reported to remain stable (or improves) at least to a mean follow-up of 6 years except in patients who already have poor renal function [50, 51]. In the series of Xu *et al.* [51], 22% of patients developed hyperchloraemic acidosis but all had significantly impaired renal function before surgery. Measurement of

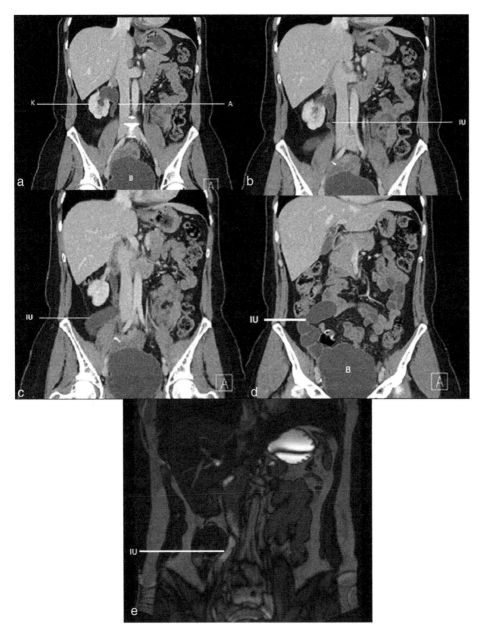

Figure 7.11 (a–d) Sagittal reconstruction of a CT IVU showing the typical appearance of a well-established ileal ureter (A, anastomosis; B, bladder; K, kidney; IU, ureter). The haustral folds have been largely lost as is normal when ileum is bathed in urine for more than 6–12 months. (e) MRI T2 urogram of a different patient showing an ileal ureter (U).

chloride and bicarbonate can be confined to those who have poor renal function.

There are inadequate data to recommend a follow-up protocol for intestinal onlay procedures or narrow tubes (appendix or Yang–Monti). They are best regarded as experimental procedures and monitored by defined protocol. Cases have been followed for as long as 10 years without evidence of renal impairment.

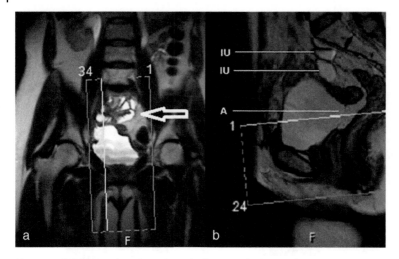

Figure 7.12 MRI urogram showing an ileal ureter which is too long It is seen with loops (a) above and (b) behind the bladder (on the scout picture, labelled IU). Despite this, renal function was stable with a CrEDTA glomerular filtration rate of 45 mL/min/1.73 m² before surgery and 53 mL/min/1.73 m² two years later at the time of this MRI. The original obstruction was caused by radiation fibrosis.

References

1 Elliott SP, McAninch JW. Ureteral injuries from external violence: the 25-year experience at San Francisco General Hospital. *J Urol.* 2003; 170(4 Pt 1): 1213–1216.

2 Wood DN, Cottrell A, Baker SC, *et al.* Recreational ketamine: from pleasure to pain. *Br J Urol Int.* 2011; 107: 1881–1884.

3 Wenske S, Olsson CA, Benson MC. Outcomes of distal ureteral reconstruction through reimplantation with psoas hitch, Boari flap, or ureteroneocystostomy for benign or malignant ureteral obstruction or injury. *Urology.* 2013; 82(1): 231–236.

4 Anderson JC, Hynes W. Retrocaval ureter: a case diagnosed pre-operatively and treated successfully by a plastic operation. *Br J Urol.* 1949; 21(3): 209–214.

5 Noble JG, Lee KT, Mundy AR. Transuretero-ureterostomy: a review of 253 cases. *Br J Urol.* 1997; 79: 20–23.

6 Norgaard JP, Dorflinger T, Gjode P, Djurhuus JC. The hydrodynamic consequences of transuretero-ureterostomia. *Urol Res.* 1987; 15(5): 277–279.

7 Mauck RJ, Hudak SJ, Terlecki RP, Morey AF. Central role of Boari bladder flap and downward nephropexy in upper ureteral reconstruction. *J Urol.* 2011; 186(4): 1345–1349.

8 Goel A, Dalela D. Options in the management of tuberculous ureteric stricture. *Indian J Urol.* 2008; 24(3): 376–381.

9 Badmos KB, Popoola AA, Buhari MO, Abdulkadir AY. Ureteric schistosomiasis with obstructive uropathy. *J Coll Physicians Surg Pak.* 2009; 19(7): 456–458.

10 Bazeed MA, Ashamalla A, Abd-Alrazek AA, Ghoneim M, Badr M. Management of bilharzial strictures of the lower ureter. *Urol Int.* 1982; 37(1): 19–25.

11 Routh JC, Tollefson MK, Ashley RA, Husmann DA. Iatrogenic ureteral injury: can adult repair techniques be used on children? *J Pediatr Urol.* 2009; 5(1): 53–55.

12 Petterson S, Aamot P, Brynger H, Johansson S, Nilson AE, Ranch T. Extracorporeal renal surgery, autotransplantation and calicovesicostomy for renal pelvic and ureteric tumours. *Scand J Urol Nephrol.* 1981; 60(Suppl): 33–35.

13 Tran G, Ramaswamy K, Chi T, Meng M, Freise C, Stoller ML. Laparoscopic nephrectomy with autotransplantation: safety, efficacy and long-term durability. *J Urol.* 2015; 194(3): 738–743.

14 Cowan NG, Banerji JS, Johnston RB, *et al.* Renal Autotransplantation: 27-year experience at 2 institutions. *J Urol.* 2015; 194(5): 1357–1361.

15 Dagash H, Sen S, Chacko J, *et al.* The appendix as ureteral substitute: a report of 10 cases. *J Pediatr Urol.* 2008; 4(1): 14–19.

16 Duty BD, Kreshover JE, Richstone L, Kavoussi LR. Review of appendiceal onlay flap in the management of complex ureteric strictures in six patients. *BJU Int.* 2015; 115(2): 282–287.

17 Castellan M, Gosalbez R. Ureteral replacement using the Yang–Monti principle: long-term follow-up. *Urology.* 2006; 67(3): 476–479.

18 Smith TG III,, Gettman M, Lindberg G, Napper C, Pearle MS, Cadeddu JA. Ureteral replacement using porcine small intestine submucosa in a porcine model. *Urology.* 2002; 60(5): 931–934.

19 El Assmy A, El Hamid MA, Hafez AT. Urethral replacement: a comparison between small intestinal submucosa grafts and spontaneous regeneration. *BJU Int.* 2004; 94(7): 1132–1135.

20 El Hakim A, Marcovich R, Chiu KY, Lee BR, Smith AD. First prize: ureteral segmental replacement revisited. *J Endourol.* 2005; 19(9): 1069–1074.

21 Shi JG, Fu WJ, Wang XX, *et al.* Tissue engineering of ureteral grafts by seeding urothelial differentiated hADSCs onto biodegradable ureteral scaffolds. *J Biomed Mater Res A.* 2012; 100(10): 2612–2622.

22 Badawy AA, Abolyosr A, Saleem MD, Abuzeid AM. Buccal mucosa graft for ureteral stricture substitution: initial experience. *Urology.* 2010; 76(4): 971–975.

23 Zhang F, Sones WD, Guo M, *et al.* Reconstruction of ureteral defects with microvascular vein grafts in a rat

model. *J Reconstr Microsurg.* 2001; 17(3): 179–183.

24 Acosta-Miranda AM, Milner J, Turk TMT. The FECal Double-J: a simplifed approach in the management of encrusted and retained ureteral stents. *J Endourol.* 2015; 23(3): 409–415.

25 Lange D, Bidnur S, Hoag N, Chew BH. Ureteral stent-associated complications: where we are and where we are going. *Nat Rev Urol.* 2015; 12(1): 17–25.

26 Chew BH, Lange D. Advances in ureteral stent development. *Curr Opin Urol.* 2016; 26(3): 277–282.

27 Klis R, Korczak-Kozakiewicz E, Denys A, Sosnowski M, Rozanski W. Relationship between urinary tract infection and self-retaining Double-J catheter colonization. *J Endourol.* 2009; 23(6): 1015–1019.

28 Farsi HM, Mosli HA, Al Zemaity MF, Bahnassy AA, Alvarez M. Bacteriuria and colonization of double-pigtail ureteral stents: long-term experience with 237 patients. *J Endourol.* 1995; 9(6): 469–472.

29 Kehinde EO, Rotimi VO, Al Awadi KA, *et al.* Factors predisposing to urinary tract infection after J ureteral stent insertion. *J Urol.* 2002; 167(3): 1334–1337.

30 Ben Meir D, Golan S, Ehrlich Y, Livne PM. Characteristics and clinical significance of bacterial colonization of ureteral double-J stents in children. *J Pediatr Urol.* 2009; 5(5): 355–358.

31 Joshi HB, Stainthorpe A, MacDonagh RP, Keeley FX Jr, Timoney AG, Barry MJ. Indwelling ureteral stents: evaluation of symptoms, quality of life and utility. *J Urol.* 2003; 169(3): 1065–1069.

32 Lee JN, Kim BS. Comparison of efficacy and bladder irritation symptoms among three different ureteral stents: a double-blind, prospective, randomized controlled trial. *Scand J Urol.* 2015; 49(3): 237–241.

33 Dellis AE, Keeley FX J, Manolas V, Skolarikos AA. Role of alpha-blockers in the treatment of stent-related symptoms:

a prospective randomized control study. *Urology.* 2014; 83(1): 56–61.

34 Sivalingam S, Streeper NM, Sehgal PD, Sninsky BC, Best SL, Nakada SY. Does combination therapy with tamsulosin and tolterodine improve ureteral stent discomfort compared with tamsulosin alone? A double-blind, randomized, controlled trial. *J Urol.* 2016; 195(2): 385–390.

35 Venkatesh R, Landman J, Minor SD, *et al.* Impact of a double-pigtail stent on ureteral peristalsis in the porcine model: initial studies using a novel implantable magnetic sensor. *J Endourol.* 2005; 19(2): 170–176.

36 Woodhouse CRJ, Wickham JEA. The effect of negative pressures in surgical drains. *Br J Urol.* 1979; 51: 597–600.

37 Elsamra SE, Leavitt DA, Motato HA, *et al.* Stenting for malignant ureteral obstruction: tandem, metal or metal–mesh stents. *Int J Urol.* 2015; 22(7): 629–636.

38 Kadlec AO, Ellimoottil CS, Greco KA, Turk TM. Five-year experience with metallic stents for chronic ureteral obstruction. *J Urol.* 2013; 190(3): 937–941.

39 Song G, Lim B, Han KS, Song SH, Park HK, Hong B. Complications after polymeric and metallic ureteral stent placements including three types of fistula. *J Endourol.* 2015; 29(4): 485–489.

40 Agrawal S, Brown CT, Bellamy EA, Kulkarni R. The thermo-expandable metallic ureteric stent: an 11-year follow-up. *BJU Int.* 2009; 103(3): 372–376.

41 Liatsikos EN, Karnabatidis D, Katsanos K, *et al.* Ureteral metal stents: 10-year experience with malignant ureteral obstruction treatment. *J Urol.* 2009; 182(6): 2613–2617.

42 Ahmed S, Sparnon SL, Savage JP, Boucaut HA, Smith AJ. Surgery of pelvi-ureteric obstruction in 101 children over one year of age. *Aust N Z J Surg.* 1986; 56: 675–680.

43 Iwaszko MR, Krambeck AE, Chow GK, Gettman MT. Transureteroureterostomy revisited: long-term surgical outcomes. *J Urol.* 2010; 183(3): 1055–1059.

44 Mure PY, Mollard P, Mouriquand P. Transureteroureterostomy in childhood and adolescence: long-term results in 69 cases. *J Urol.* 2000; 163(3): 946–948.

45 Bowsher WG, Shah PJ, Costello AJ, Tiptaft RC, Paris AM, Blandy JP. A critical appraisal of the Boari flap. *Br J Urol.* 1982; 54(6): 682–685.

46 Flatmark A, Albrechtsen D, Sodal G, Bondevik H, Jakobsen A Jr, Brekke IB. Renal autotransplantation. *World J Surg.* 1989; 13(2): 206–209.

47 Bodie B, Novick AC, Rose M, Straffon RA. Long-term results with renal autotransplantation for ureteral replacement. *J Urol.* 1986; 136(6): 1187–1189.

48 Plas E, Kretschmer G, Stackl W, Steininger R, Muhlbacher F, Pfluger H. Experience in renal autotransplantation: analysis of a clinical series. *Br J Urol.* 1996; 77(4): 518–523.

49 Azhar B, Patel S, Chadha P, Hakim N. Indications for renal autotransplant: an overview. *Exp Clin Transplant.* 2015; 13(2): 109–114.

50 Chung BI, Hamawy KJ, Zinman LN, Libertino JA. The use of bowel for ureteral replacement for complex ureteral reconstruction: long-term results. *J Urol.* 2006; 175(1): 179–183.

51 Xu YM, Feng C, Kato H, Xie H, Zhang XR. Long-term outcome of ileal ureteric replacement with an iliopsoas muscle tunnel antirefluxing technique for the treatment of long-segment ureteric strictures. *Urology.* 2016; 88: 201–206.

52 Woodhouse CRJ. *Adolescent Urology and Long-Term Outcomes.* Oxford: Wiley, 2015.

53 Woodhouse CRJ. Supra-vesical urinary diversion and ureteric re-implantation for malignant disease. *Clin Oncol.* 2010; 22: 727–732.

8

Conservative and Reconstructive Bladder Surgery

Pardeep Kumar

Introduction

The urinary bladder is fascinating in its ability to heal following trauma or surgical insult, maintain function and adapt to changes in surrounding structures. Its position in the pelvis along with the proximity to adjacent viscera makes it vulnerable to damage from radiotherapy, surgery and trauma. This chapter outlines the imaging appearances following various treatments and supplies rationale to follow-up regimens.

Extravasation

Endoscopy became commonplace in the twentieth century. All modern cystoscopes utilise an irrigant to distend the bladder and improve visualisation. A degree of transmural absorption occurs with most procedures even in the absence of bladder perforation [1]. Risk factors for increasing 'extravasation' include previous therapy and high intravesical pressure (this may be secondary to irrigant pressure or poor bladder compliance). Following anything other than the most straightforward of procedures this results in oedema in the extravesical space which can make interpretation of the pelvis difficult on imaging in the early postoperative period (Figure 8.1).

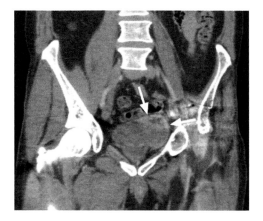

Figure 8.1 A coronal enhanced CT image in a patient who had undergone a transurethral resection of bladder tumour 48 hours previously. In the absence of any clinical perforation there is oedema of the bladder wall (arrow) and surrounding tissues in the extravesical space. Should accurate staging of the bladder wall be the aim then a pre-operative scan would have been more useful. Where this is unavailable, deferring imaging for 2 weeks is usually sufficient to allow the oedema to resolve.

Bladder Perforation

When reported in a subjective manner, bladder perforation is uncommon even during loop resection of bladder tumours (3% in a UK wide 'snapshot' audit of transurethral resection of bladder tumours, TURBT) [2]. When perforation is actively examined for

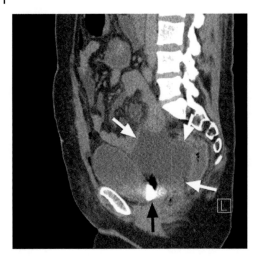

Figure 8.2 A sagittal CT in a patient who had undergone a radical hysterectomy 5 days previously. Severe abdominal pain at the time of catheter removal raised the possibility of a bladder injury. CT urogram with a catheter in situ shows a collection posterior to the bladder (white arrows). Interestingly, the balloon of the catheter appeared to sit in the defect stopping the contrast (black arrow) from passing into the posterior collection to confirming the diagnosis.

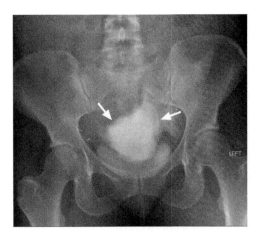

Figure 8.3 An AP pelvis radiograph 30 minutes post intravenous contrast administration in the same patient. This clearly demonstrated contrast within the collection posterior to the bladder (arrows) confirming a lower urinary tract injury. Subsequent cystoscopy showed a 5-cm vertical midline defect in the bladder which appeared to be an ischaemic injury. Both ureters were intact. At laparotomy a layered closure was undertaken and omentum interposed between the bladder and vaginal stump.

with a cystogram post resection it is detected in up to 58% of cases [3–5]. Clearly, the clinical relevance of perforation is dependent on the size of the defect as well as its position – dome and posterior wall injuries resulting in communication with the intraperitoneal cavity are likely to require more than just prolonged catheter drainage (Figures 8.2, 8.3 and 8.4).

Extraperitoneal bladder injuries are usually managed conservatively. Small injuries from biopsy forceps appear to heal satisfactorily after 24 hours of catheter drainage and antibiotics [4]. Larger defects and those in bladders where healing may be impaired (irradiation) or where intravesical pressures may be higher than normal (chronic urinary retention) may benefit from longer periods of drainage [5]. Injury from blunt trauma requires still longer

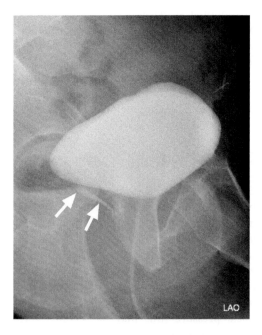

Figure 8.4 A lateral view at cystogram in the same patient 6 weeks post repair. A persistent vesico-vaginal fistula is demonstrated (the vaginal contrast is shown by arrows). Cystoscopy demonstrated a pinhole defect at the inferior aspect of the bladder closure. A soft-tipped hydrophilic guide wire passed into this showed communication with the vaginal vault. This was successfully repaired transvaginally 3 months following the initial hysterectomy.

periods of catheterisation, particularly where there are associated bony injuries. Up to 25% of trauma patients managed with catheter drainage alone develop complications and many experts advocate operative repair of these if possible [6, 7].

Bladder injuries at the time of TURB present two immediate problems. The first is the need to manage the perforation and exclude concurrent injuries to adjacent viscera, the second is to deal with the risk of intra-abdominal tumour seeding. Small extraperitoneal perforations do not seem to infer a marked increase in tumour seeding and pelvic recurrence [5]. Tumours confined to the lamina propria (pTa) appear to have little risk of spread even with intraperitoneal perforation [8]. Locally advanced disease, however, is associated with a risk of seeding. Where possible, laparotomy, washout and bladder repair is advocated (Figure 8.5). No role for adjuvant chemotherapy in this group has been established [9].

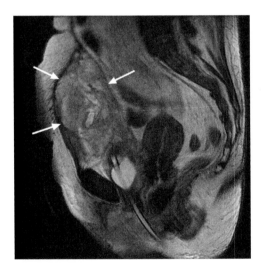

Figure 8.5 A coronal T2-weighted MRI image in a patient who had undergone a transurethral resection of bladder tumour (TURBT) complicated by perforation. Tumour seeding occurred (arrows) with local invasion into the rectus sheath. Anterior exenteration with en bloc removal of the anterior abdominal wall was required to obtain clear surgical margins. A skin-sparing approach facilitated reconstruction with biological mesh.

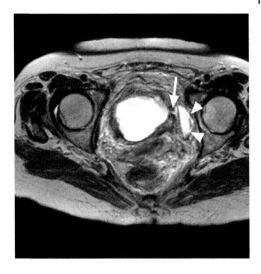

Figure 8.6 T2 axial MRI image showing a thick-walled bladder with an extraperitoneal perforation on the left lateral wall. The defect is shown by an arrow; a small extravesical collection by the arrowheads. There is surrounding oedema which extends posteriorly to the rectum as well as encircling the bladder. An unrecognised perforation at the time of TURBT allowed intravesical mitomycin used postoperatively to escape into the pelvis. Severe immediate pain at the time of instillation persisted until anterior exenteration was carried out. Findings at surgery included obliteration of normal tissue planes in the pelvis and a dense fibrosis extending up into the retroperitoneum.

Intravesical mitomycin C is currently recommended in the immediate postoperative setting as a means of reducing local recurrence rates following endoscopic bladder cancer surgery. As outlined earlier, many patients have unrecognised small perforations at the time of TURBT [3–5]. It is therefore unsurprising that a proportion of patients develop the devastating complication of mitomycin extravasation (Figure 8.6) [10, 11].

Reconstruction Following Ureteric Injury and Partial Cystectomy

Both benign and malignant conditions of the bladder can sometimes be managed with

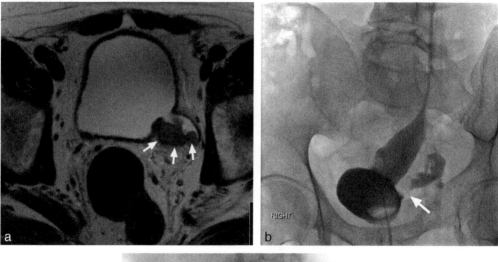

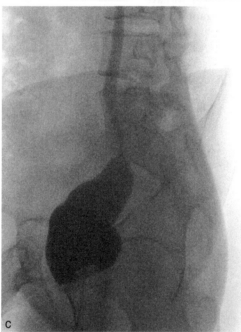

Figure 8.7 (a) T2 axial MRI image showing a solid tumour lying within a left-sided bladder diverticulum. This squamous cell cancer was locally advanced and impinging on the ipsilateral ureter. Partial cystectomy and ureteric re-implantation into a Boari flap achieved clear surgical margins. (b) Cystogram 1 week later in the same patient. A persistent leak (arrow) at the inferior portion of the bladder closure was managed by a further 2 weeks of catheterisation. (c) Cystogram taken on the day of catheter removal. The leak had resolved. Despite initial functional volumes being only 150 mL per void, at 6 weeks this had risen to 300 mL.

partial cystectomy, with ureteric re-implantation where required. If enough healthy bladder is available, patients can expect to regain near-normal capacity over 6–8 weeks. Should the pelvis have been irradiated, the bladder may not regain normal capacity and consideration is given to a concurrent augmentation procedure.

Follow-up schedules for the reconstruction itself are tailored to the individual situation.

In most patients, an early ultrasound (US) following removal of all catheters, drains and stents acts as a baseline for future examinations. It also serves to highlight the early complication of stenosis at the re-implantation site. The relationship of any upper tract dilatation to bladder volume should be noted. A dilated renal pelvis with a full bladder is normal with a refluxing anastomosis but should be seen to resolve or improve following voiding [12].

The effect of pelvic radiation on the urinary tract can be severe and progressive. Over time short strictures become long ones; unilateral disease becomes bilateral. Because of this, follow-up is prolonged after reconstruction in this scenario. US

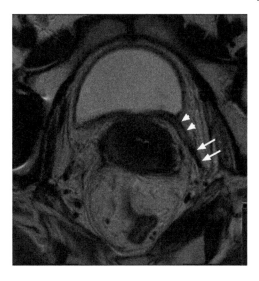

Figure 8.9 T2 axial MRI image showing a fibrotic, strictured segment of left ureter (arrows) in a 30-year-old woman 1 year post external beam and brachytherapy for cervical cancer. The most distal ureter is more normal in calibre but still thickened (arrowheads). The adjacent uterus shows typical post treatment change. The proximal ureter was dilated; at the time of surgery, fibrotic change was noted over a much longer segment of ureter necessitating a ureteric re-implantation using a psoas hitch.

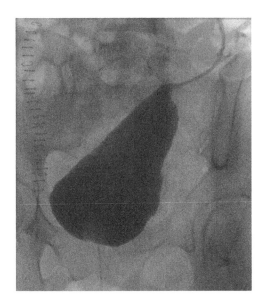

Figure 8.8 Cystogram at the time of catheter removal 2 weeks following excision of a 20-cm pelvic schwannoma. The Boari flap in this case extended to the upper–mid ureteric junction. With downward nephropexy and a large capacity bladder it is possible to carry out replacement of the entire ureter utilising this technique [14]. The appearance of a Boari flap is variable; in this image it looks as if the 'flap' is in fact just a psoas hitch of the bladder; in Figure 8.7 it has almost the typical 'rabbit's ear' appearance, while in Figure 7.9 it looks like a narrow, irregular tube. All of these are variations of normal. Source: Mauck *et al.* (2011) [14]. Reproduced with permission of Elsevier.

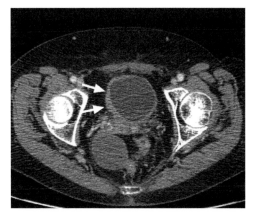

Figure 8.10 This enhanced axial CT image shows eccentric bladder thickening in a 79-year-old patient 3 years post radical radiotherapy for bladder cancer. Bilateral hydroureter was present secondary to lower ureteric fibrosis. Eventually she underwent supravesical diversion into an ileal conduit. Her bladder remains under cystoscopic surveillance and has contracted down to around 50 mL in capacity.

remains the investigation of choice and should be carried out annually in the absence of signs of progression such as flank pain and haematuria.

At the end of the nineteenth century Boari described a procedure to reconstruct the lower ureter utilising a bladder flap (Figures 8.7 and 8.8 on page 104) [13, 14]. Satisfactory bladder capacity is usually estimated at pre-operative cystoscopy (see also Chapter 7).

The Irradiated Bladder

Neoadjuvant chemotherapy followed by radiotherapy is a recognised treatment for muscle invasive bladder cancer with equivalent outcomes to cystectomy in highly selected patients [15]. Imaging of the bladder following this can be difficult to interpret even years following completion of treatment. Bladder wall thickening because of fibrosis can be asymmetric, mimicking appearances of recurrent disease (Figures 8.9, 8.10 on page 105 and 8.11).

Complications After Posterior Exenteration

The bladder and lower ureters remain at risk during posterior exenteration for gynaecological and colorectal malignancy. Many of these patients undergo pre-operative radiotherapy to downstage their tumours. This

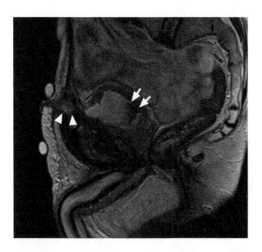

Figure 8.11 Sagittal view of the abdomen and pelvis of a patient who has undergone radical radiotherapy for high risk prostate cancer and subsequent high dose rate (HDR) brachytherapy for recurrence. He developed severe pelvic radiation disease with radionecrosis of the prostatic urethra and pelvic sepsis complicated by symphisis pubis osteomyelitis. He eventually required supravesical diversion into an ileal conduit. One year postoperatively he developed a pyocysitis prompting this MRI. Layering of material in the remnant bladder (arrows) is seen on the sagittal T2 image, along with tracking anteriorly via his previous suprapubic catheter site (arrowheads) which required drainage and antibiotics. He went on to completion cystectomy after resolution of this bout of pyocystis.

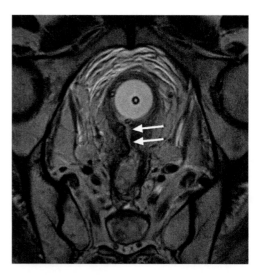

Figure 8.12 Axial T2-weighted MRI in a patient who has undergone salvage surgery in the setting of anastomotic recurrence following anterior resection of rectal tumour. Pre-operative radiotherapy downstaged the recurrence and an R0 resection was achieved. Unfortunately, an area on the posterior aspect of the bladder and lower left ureter necrosed in the postoperative period resulting in the fistula demonstrated in this image (arrows). There is a Foley catheter in the bladder. Ureteric continuity was restored via a 'rendezvous' type procedure – a simultaneous antegrade and retrograde ureteric stent placement. The bladder was kept empty for a 6-week period while the fistula healed. The patient remains stent dependent.

often causes medial deviation of the lower ureters as they are drawn in by the resulting fibrotic process. Where preservation of the anterior structures is attempted, early complications including stricture and fistulation may occur (Figure 8.12).

Conclusions

The bladder is a forgiving organ. It can be changed in shape and position and it will still perform its role in the safe storage and evacuation of urine. Long-term follow-up is often required to watch for the progressive effects of fibrosis and radiation. Early complications (in particular, leaks) are best imaged by a contrast cystogram, CT urogram or CT cystogram. Although more expensive, MRI shows perforation very well and can give much additional information about pelvic pathology. In the longer term, imaging is central to follow-up, with US key for the detection of upper tract dilatation. As in other locations, a suitable MRI generally has the best soft tissue contrast, though CT is also useful for the detection of local complications and recurrent tumour.

References

1 Hultén JO, Sundström GS. Extra vascular absorption of irrigating fluid during TURP. The role of transmural bladder pressure as the driving pressure gradient. *Br J Urol.* 1990; 65(1): 39–42.

2 Gan C, Patel A, Fowler S, Catto J, Rosario D, O'Brien T. Snapshot of transurethral resection of bladder tumors in the United Kingdom Audit (STUKA). *BJU Int.* 2013; 112(7): 930–935.

3 El Hayek OR, Coelho RF, Dall'oglio MF, *et al.* Evaluation of the incidence of bladder perforation after transurethral bladder tumor resection in a residency setting. *J Endourol.* 2009; 23(7): 1183–1186.

4 Sigler LJ, Addonizio JC, Fernandez R, Schutte H. Incidence and treatment of bladder perforation following bladder biopsy. *Urology.* 1985; 26(1): 10–11.

5 Balbay MD, Cimentepe E, Unsal A, Bayrak O, Koç A, Akbulut Z. The actual incidence of bladder perforation following transurethral bladder surgery. *J Urol.* 2005; 174(6): 2260–2262.

6 Kotkin L, Koch MO. Morbidity associated with nonoperative management of extraperitoneal bladder injuries. *J Trauma.* 1995; 38(6): 895–898.

7 Corriere JN Jr, Sandler CM. Mechanisms of injury, patterns of extravasation and management of extraperitoneal bladder rupture due to blunt trauma. *J Urol.* 1988; 139(1): 43–44.

8 Golan S, Baniel J, Lask D, Livne PM, Yossepowitch O. Transurethral resection of bladder tumor complicated by perforation requiring open surgical repair: clinical characteristics and oncological outcomes. *BJU Int.* 2011; 107(7): 1065–1068.

9 Mydlo JH, Weinstein R, Shah S, Solliday M, Macchia RJ. Long-term consequences from bladder perforation and/or violation in the presence of transitional cell carcinoma: results of a small series and a review of the literature. *J Urol.* 1999; 161(4): 1128–1132.

10 Elmamoun MH, Christmas TJ, Woodhouse CR. Destruction of the bladder by single dose Mitomycin C for low-stage transitional cell carcinoma (TCC): avoidance, recognition, management and consent. *BJU Int.* 2014; 113(5b): E34–E38.

11 Filson CP, Montgomery JS, Dailey SM, *et al.* Complications associated with single-dose, perioperative mitomycin C for patients undergoing bladder tumor resection. *Urol Oncol.* 2014; 32(1): 40.e1–e8.

12 Wenske S, Olsson CA, Benson MC. Outcomes of distal ureteral reconstruction through reimplantation with psoas hitch, Boari flap, or ureteroneocystostomy for benign or malignant ureteral obstruction or injury. *Urology*. 2013; 82(1): 231–236.

13 Dunfield VM. Boari operation in case of solitary kidney: treatment of obstruction of solitary ureter following hysterectomy. *AMA Arch Surg*. 1955; 70(3): 328–332.

14 Mauck RJ, Hudak SJ, Terlecki RP, Morey AF. Central role of Boari bladder flap and downward nephropexy in upper ureteral reconstruction. *J Urol*. 2011; 186(4): 1345–1349.

15 James ND, Hussain SA, Hall E, *et al*; BC2001 Investigators. Radiotherapy with or without chemotherapy in muscle-invasive bladder cancer. *N Engl J Med*. 2012; 366(16): 1477–1488.

9

Bladder Augmentation in Children

Paddy Dewan and Padma Rao

Introduction

A bowel segment was first used for bladder augmentation on 12 May 1898 by Rutkowski from Krakow. Many technical variations of the detubularised isolated bowel loop have since been clinically applied. The indications for enterocystoplasties have expanded, and various bowel segments such as ileum [1, 2], ileum plus caecum [3, 4] caecum [5, 6] and sigmoid colon [7, 8] have been shown to produce comparable functional results [9, 10].

In the recent past these developments have been supported by anticholinergic drugs, clean intermittent catheterisation (CIC) [11], creation of catheterisable channels [12, 13] and advanced management of bladder outlet resistance by endoscopic augmentation techniques [14, 15] or the use of artificial urinary sphincter systems [16]. There are risks and complications related to the technique employed, the nature of the underlying bladder pathology and the generality of bladder enlargement.

The Procedures

Augmentation with Ileum or Colon

The standard procedure for making the bladder larger and reducing its intrinsic pressure is to open it sagittally or coronally and put in a gusset of bowel. The operations are given the general title of 'clam' cystoplasty.

Gastrocystoplasty

The problems generated by the use of ileum prompted experimental and then clinical use of stomach as a patch. Extensive work has been carried out on the risks of gastrocystoplasty [17–20]. Possible benefits of acid secretion in the urine are confounded with adverse effects of the acid urine, with marked symptoms from acid in the bladder and urethra the most important complication in gastrocystoplasty patients [21]. As long-term follow-up is still lacking in humans, only studies in rats indicate the risk of metaplasia in both the adjacent urothelium and the incorporated segment of gastric mucosa [17], warranting lifelong follow-up for gastrocystoplasty patients. Nevertheless, for selected patients, and children in particular, there is increasing evidence that the majority of reported gastrocystoplasties improve urodynamic bladder function and clinical behaviour of the patients [22, 23]. This success, in rather difficult clinical situations, together with a reduced overall risk has to be appreciated, but, all the same, the procedure has limited applicability.

Seromuscular Cystoplasty

As many of the complications of cystoplasty are caused by the mucosa of the bowel segment employed, there have been several attempts to use de-epithelialised segments [24]. Unfortunately, there has been limited success because of the slow growth of

Radiology and Follow-up of Urologic Surgery, First Edition. Edited by Christopher Woodhouse and Alex Kirkham.
© 2018 John Wiley & Sons Ltd. Published 2018 by John Wiley & Sons Ltd.

urothelium which allows inflammation and fibrosis of the patch, resulting in shrinkage. Also, calculi formation and regeneration of the bowel mucosa occur.

Auto-augmentation

The removal of a patch of detrusor muscle, or incision of the detrusor, was first described by Huggins in 1931. Several groups reported good results with this technique in a number of children [25] and adults. In our laboratory, in a sheep model, auto-augmentation covered with omentum resulted in no long-term augmenting effect [26, 27]. In the largest series to date, Stohrer *et al.* [28] reported their experience from a spinal cord injury/disease centre in Germany. Forty-three patients with various spinal cord pathologies were managed with auto-augmentation. Much more consistent and impressive changes in bladder storage were found than in paediatric series. Mean bladder capacity went from 121 mL (range 20–300 mL) to 406 mL (range 200–600 mL), while compliance rose from 7.1 (14–30) to 29.3 (range 12–62).

Auto-augmentation alone is not applicable to patients with a small contracted bladder (Figure 9.1), bladder exstrophy or a markedly trabeculated bladder (Figure 9.2). Auto-augmentation backed by either demucosalised stomach or colon has proved successful. In particular, the backing reduces the risk of adverse changes to the auto-augmented bladder in the long term. Dewan *et al.* [29–31] used seromuscular segments from stomach or colon first in a sheep model and then in patients with good results. Other backings have been attempted, but have not endured the test of time. Tissue engineering techniques may be used in the future.

Uretero-cystoplasty

Reconstruction of the urinary tract would ideally be carried out with urothelial tissues. Surplus ureter is sometimes available. The ideal patient is one with a non-functioning kidney with high grade vesico-ureteric reflux that is concurrently resolved during the

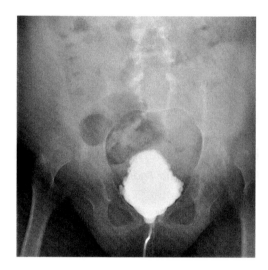

Figure 9.1 Contrast study outlining a small volume, irregular trabeculated bladder which is unsuitable for auto-augmentation because of the need for an adequate urothelial diverticulum formation, as is the case for most exstrophy bladders; the latter would show a flat bladder base. Incidental note is also made of spina bifida and severe bilateral hip dysplasia with bilateral hip dislocation.

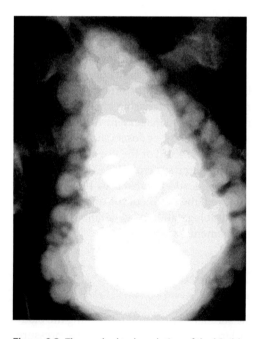

Figure 9.2 The marked trabeculation of the bladder suggests that techniques that involve auto-augmentation would be difficult.

procedure. It is particularly appropriate for children less than 2 years old in whom clams with any bowel segment are best avoided.

Originally, both the renal pelvis and the megaureter were thought necessary to ensure an adequate increase in bladder volume. More recent studies have shown that the lower two-thirds of a dilated ureter provide a considerable increase in bladder capacity, allowing for preservation of the ipsilateral kidney. Several techniques have been reported. Importantly, it can be carried out via an extraperitoneal approach which avoids the risk of contamination of existing ventriculo-peritoneal shunts and facilitates subsequent peritoneal dialysis. Also, in the female, there is no pedicle to interfere with a caesarean section if required in later years. The extraperitoneal approach can also be used to perform a combination of uretero-cystoplasty and the trans-uretero-ureterostomy, by anastomosing the two ureters retroperitoneally [32]. The ability to join the two ureters via a lateral approach is understandable by noting that ureters can be seen overlapping on a cystogram (Figure 9.3). Thus, the benefits of the extraperitoneal approach can be achieved while preserving the function of the ipsilateral kidney (Figure 9.4).

Both ultrasound (US) (Figure 9.5) and cystography (Figure 9.6) can be used to assess the adequacy of the ureter for bladder augmentation.

Although uretero-cystoplasty may not provide the same increase in bladder volume as can be expected from enterocystoplasty, intra-abdominal, bowel mucosal and nutritional consequences of standard cystoplasty are avoided. Mucus is not formed by urothelium, most children can void normally and have a low incidence of infection. Stones are very rare. It is presumed that there will be no increased risk of malignancy.

Clinical Follow-up

The clinical follow-up for bladder augmentation relates to the component parts that are used for the bladder enlargement, continence and renal status. The investigation of the bladder pertains to its function, the lining of the bladder and the metabolic impact on the patient of the segment used to augment the bladder. It should be standard practice to follow-up patients who have had urinary tract reconstructions for life. In the case of children, appropriate arrangements must be made for transition to adult care.

The ureteric catheters are usually removed at 10 days. The suprapubic catheter is clamped at 3 weeks for trials of voiding. A patient with an augmented bladder should always be expected to need CIC, accepting that patients who do not have a neuropathic bladder may be able to void spontaneously. CIC is started if proper voiding is not

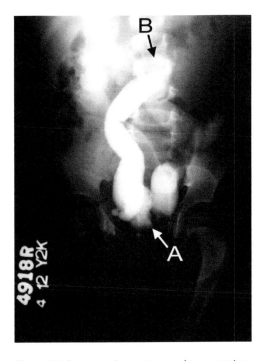

Figure 9.3 Pre-operative cystogram demonstrating small volume, trabeculated bladder (A), and high grade, bilateral vesicoureteric reflux outlining dilated tortuous ureters. The upper ureters can be seen to overlap (B), indicating that the ipsilateral and contralateral ureters can be joined via a lateral approach.

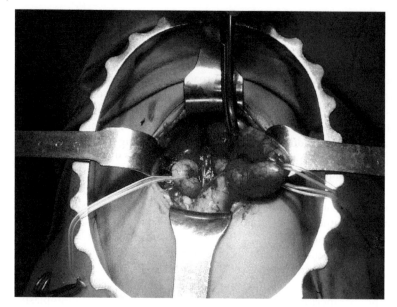

Figure 9.4 At operation (same patient as in figure 9.3), through a left lateral wound, in the extraperitoneal plane, both ureters can be seen with slings around them, the left on right and the right on the left of the image.

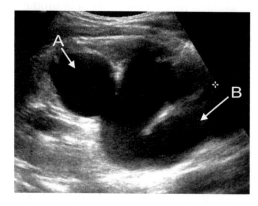

Figure 9.5 The upper ureter and pelvis can be assessed with an ultrasound (US) of the upper tract; in this case the dilated calyces (A) and dilated ureter (B) are noted, and help to gauge the suitability of the ureter for uretero-cystoplasty.

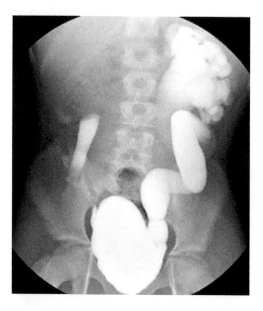

Figure 9.6 The existence of vesico-ureteric reflux on a cystogram also allows for the size of the ureters and the suitability of the ureter for uretero-cystoplasty to be assessed.

established, a process that should be facilitated by training prior to surgery. If a continent stoma is formed as part of the augmentation, the stomal catheter is removed and CIC commenced via the Mitrofanoff conduit. The suprapubic catheter remains in place until CIC is well established, then, on the day of the removal of the suprapubic catheter, an indwelling catheter is left in situ via either the urethra or Mitrofanoff overnight, and overnight for the next 4 weeks.

A cystogram to understand the initial anatomy is appropriately performed prior to the removal of the suprapubic catheter. US of the upper urinary tract can be deferred until 4 weeks after the procedure, provided the clinical course is satisfactory. Any suggestion of sepsis should prompt an early US to check the kidneys and review for a leak.

A urodynamic study is deferred until 3 months after the procedure, when the need for continuing anticholinergic medication can be considered; in some cases it may need to be continued, noting that some of the improvement in bladder performance occurs over time because of decreased work hypertrophy of the native bladder.

A suggestion of late or early leak from the bladder is investigated with a combination of radiological techniques. However, small leaks can be hard to find and may not be bothersome; investigation must be governed by the clinical situation.

Antibiotic prophylaxis in the first 4 weeks is advocated, but thereafter, other than when there is *febrile* sepsis, positive urine cultures should be managed with improved bladder drainage and increased fluid throughput.

Importantly, when bowel mucosa is incorporated into the bladder, the patient and family should be made aware of the risk of bladder perforation.

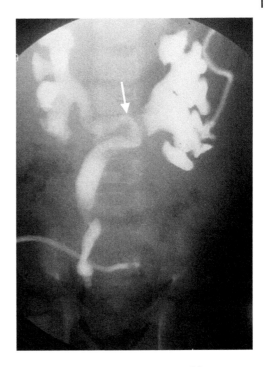

Figure 9.7 The postoperative image of the anastomosis between the left and right ureters (arrow) can be achieved via either a nephrostomy or, most usually, a transvesical ureteric catheter.

Postoperative Imaging

In the postoperative period, imaging is aimed at ensuring the bladder is water-tight, the upper tracts are stable and there are no leaks from any anastomoses (Figure 9.7). In the long term, imaging aims to monitor for complications in the asymptomatic patient.

A cystogram is usually performed at 3 weeks to 1 month post surgery, prior to the instigation of CIC. If an upper tract anastomosis has been performed as part of the procedure, a contrast study via either a nephrostomy or ureteric catheter is undertaken, usually prior to the study of the bladder, and most often at about 10 days postoperatively (Figure 9.7).

In patients who have had bladder augmentation as part of a secondary closure of bladder exstrophy, with a bladder neck repair, a contrast study of the urethra is also undertaken.

Video-urodynamic studies are usually reserved until at least 3 months after the procedure and, depending on clinical progress, would appropriately be repeated 1 year after the bladder enlargement (Figures 9.8, 9.9 and 9.10).

US is the best investigation for long-term monitoring and can be compared with pre-operative studies. The initial study should be at 3 months and then according to progress, but certainly annually in the first instance.

Other radiological studies may be required. Renal status and function are assessed biochemically, with nuclear medicine investigations if needed. Stone disease or suspected bladder perforation can be assessed by CT (Figure 9.11) or contrast radiography (Figure 9.12).

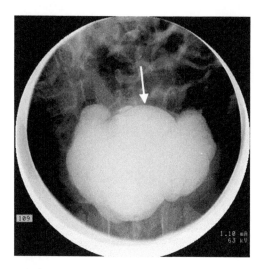

Figure 9.8 A cystogram of the bladder after uretero-cystoplasty demonstrates the mid portion of the bladder, formed by the ureter, as a smooth dome-shaped connection (arrow) between the two lateral portions that are the native bladder, which was seen to expand as the lateral bladder components contracted during a urodynamic study.

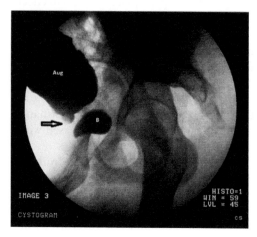

Figure 9.10 The hourglass arrangement of the bladder (B) and ileal patch (Aug) can occur from insufficient incision of the bladder, with contraction of the anastomosis (arrowed).

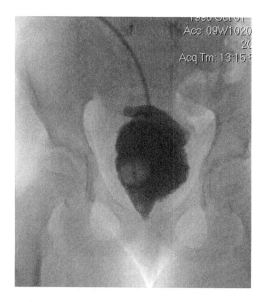

Figure 9.9 The irregular bladder of an ileo-caecal augment can be seen in the early postoperative contrast study via a suprapubic catheter that is performed to exclude a leak prior to removal of the suprapubic catheter.

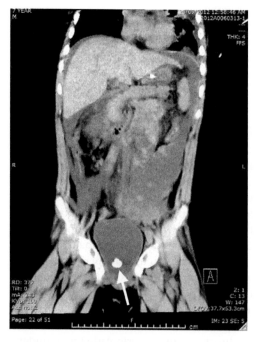

Figure 9.11 CT scanning has become the mainstream investigation for calculi in adults, but should be used sparingly in children because of the high radiation burden. Coronal CT image of the abdomen and pelvis demonstrates a bladder stone (arrow).

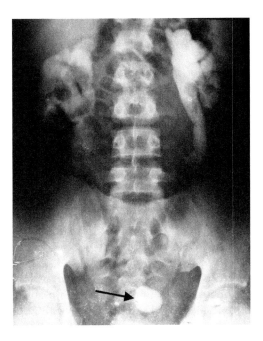

Figure 9.12 Image from an intravenous urogram demonstrates the presence of a large bladder calculus (arrow), best seen during the early phase of the study prior to contrast filling the urinary bladder.

Complications of Enterocystoplasty

Metabolic and Electrolyte Disorders

(see also Chapter 11)

Ion absorption and the subsequent development of metabolic abnormality are affected by the type of gut segment used and the amount of absorptive surface exposed to urine. Electrolytes move across and between the gut mucosal cells by both active and passive transport systems. Chloride and ammonium are selectively reabsorbed from the urine resulting in hyperchloraemic metabolic acidosis [33]. Water moves between the cell junctions according to an osmotic gradient, affected by the tightness of the cell junctions. Moving distally down the bowel segments, the cell junctions allow less and less water loss, such that the colon is rather impermeable to water. In contrast, the loose cell junctions of the jejunum allow massive water loss, contributing to the serious metabolic complications demonstrated in patients with jejunal conduits.

Early reports of metabolic complications after enterocystoplasty implicated pre-existing renal insufficiency [34]. In a large series of both paediatric and adult patients followed long-term after augmentation with ileum, colon, caecum or tubular sigmoid, Mitchell and Piser [35] reported mild hyperchloraemia developing in all groups regardless of type of bowel segment used. However, acidosis only developed in those patients with renal insufficiency.

In a prospective study of 48 paediatric and adult enterocystoplasty patients, Nurse and Mundy [36] measured electrolyte absorption in the augmented bladders after intravenous administration of radio-labelled isotopes. They reported hyperchloraemia in 26% of patients with ileo-cystoplasties. All patients had abnormal blood gases, with the majority demonstrating metabolic acidosis with respiratory compensation. There was a trend toward decreased reabsorption with time after surgery in patients who had undergone reconstruction with ileum, but not in patients with ileo-caecal segments. The authors suggest that this may reflect villous atrophy in the ileal segment, as previously described in ileal conduits and continent reservoirs [37]. However, the data are not serial measurements on the same patient and no conclusions regarding the natural history of the gut mucosa in each patient can be reached from this study. Although increased time of exposure of gut mucosa to urine would seem to increase the risk for metabolic changes, they found that augmentation cystoplasties had no greater risk of metabolic abnormality than that seen with bowel conduits that drain continuously [36].

Stones

Urinary tract calculi are a potentially serious complication of enterocystoplasty. Pyelonephritis, multiple operations and even death are reported in two large series addressing urolithiasis after bladder augmentation in children [38]. Adult series of enterocystoplasty have either not mentioned calculi as a complication or have found a low incidence in their patient population [39]. The reported incidence of stone formation after augmentation in children ranges widely from 3% to 52% [38, 40].

The aetiology of stone formation in patients with urine stored in bowel is multifactorial (see Chapter 11). Both the underlying condition of the patient and the type of urinary reservoir are relevant. Studies of the incidence of stones in reconstructed patients do not always take these factors into account and not all of the predisposing factors are present in patients with clam augmentations.

Metabolic abnormalities may be unrelated to the reconstruction. Palmer *et al.* [41] analysed 24-hour urine tests in their stone-formers and found hypocitraturia to be the only abnormality. The children were treated with oral potassium citrate and no recurrence of urolithiasis was noted. Post-augmentation upper tract stones occurred in 3 of 26 stone-formers (12%), with no patients in the series admitting to pre-augmentation urolithiasis [41].

Within the reservoir the surface area of intestine is less with a clam than with complete bladder replacements. Therefore, predisposing factors related to bowel are lessened. In those with gastric or ureteric clams stones are very rare.

Persistent bacteriuria is a leading cause of stone formation after enterocystoplasty. Bladder stone composition after augmentation with bowel in children is predominately apatite struvite and ammonium urate. Struvite was the major component in ileo-cystoplasty stones while ileo-caecocystoplasties had the highest composition of ammonium urate stones in the series reported by Blyth *et al.* [38].

Urine stasis predisposes many patients to infection and subsequent stones. Urine is commonly retained in augmented bladders because of abnormal bladder contour and inefficient drainage. This situation is worsened by increasing bladder capacity and less frequent intermittent catheterisation by

some patients. The data of Blyth *et al.* [38] suggest that Mitrofanoff drainage may be a further risk factor for stone formation, with one-third of their reported stone patients emptying via an appendico-vesicostomy. They found urinary tract calculi in 30% of 87 children with bladder augmentation or substitution. The majority had undergone sigmoid colocystoplasty and almost half emptied through a Mitrofanoff catheterisable conduit [38]. Stones recurred in 20%.

The use of small drainage catheters and the dependent position of the bladder relative to the catheterisable channel may result in poor drainage of mucus, which can be seen on US (Figure 9.13). Retention of mucus in the augmented bladder is common and appears to contribute to infection and stone formation in some patients. Daily irrigation with 300 ml of tap water was shown to decrease the incidence of stone formation in children with bladder augmentation [42].

In a large series of bladder augmentation in children and young adults, Hendren and Hendren [40] reported stones as their most common postoperative complication, occurring in 23 of 129 patients (18%). Almost 75% of the stones occurred after caecal cystoplasty and half occurred on staples of an anti-reflux nipple. Non-absorbable

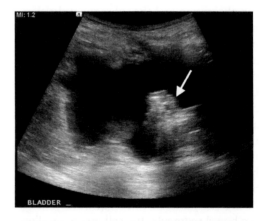

Figure 9.13 An US can be used to find calculi in the renal tract. The US image demonstrates echogenic mucus adherent to the bladder wall (arrow), often the forme fruste of calculi. Absence of an acoustic shadow confirms that it is not (yet) a stone.

materials should not be used in urinary tract reconstructions. However, even absorbable staples may precipitate stones. Palmer *et al.* [41] found absorbable staple 'ghosts' within bladder calculi as well as calculi attached to metal staples.

The background incidence of reservoir stones in patients with an ileal clam and no other relevant factors is probably about 3% at 4 years. Attention to stone prevention is essential. Antibiotic prophylaxis is not recommended except in patients with vesico-ureteric reflux. Inhibition of the urease reaction by acetohydroxamic acid therapy (where available) has not been adequately tested [38]. Diligent catheterisation with thorough bladder emptying must be reinforced regularly. Recurrent stone formation is common and is an indication to change bladder management.

Perforation

Bladder perforation after augmentation is a rare but life-threatening event. It can be diagnosed on CT and MRI (Figure 9.14), but US, which is the appropriate initial investigation,

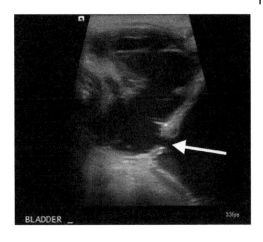

Figure 9.15 A bladder leak after augmentation may have variable clinical presentation and in severe cases the patient may present with generalised peritonitis. The US image demonstrates the presence of a defect in the bladder wall (arrow) confirming the presence of a perforation.

can also be diagnostic (Figures 9.15 and 9.16). Delay in diagnosis because of lack of normal sensation in many patients undergoing enterocystoplasty, combined with lack of suspicion on the part of managing physicians, has resulted in death in some patients [43].

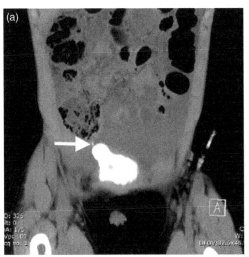
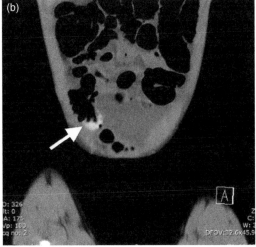

Figure 9.14 (a) When a bladder leak does occur, which is relatively rare, it usually occurs from the junction of the bladder and bowel mucosa, and can be difficult to diagnose, usually requiring CT scanning. Coronal CT cystogram image of the abdomen and pelvis demonstrates a small beak of contrast emanating from the bladder dome (arrow) confirming the site of the leak. (b) Coronal CT image of the same patient as in (a) taken more anteriorly demonstrates a small collection of contrast around the caecal pole (arrow) confirming the presence of the bladder leak.

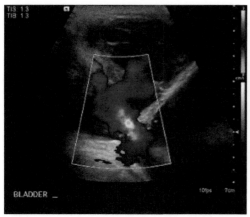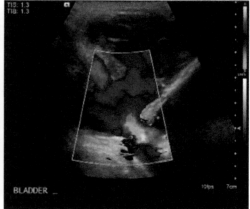

Figure 9.16 (a,b) Doppler study of the perforation of the bladder demonstrates flow from urine moving from within the bladder into the extravesical collection (red flare), with the flow reversing (shown by the reduction of the red flare in the extra vesical collection) with increasing abdominal pressure confirming the frank perforation. Cystogram alone may give a false negative image even when other modalities confirm that a leak is present.

The aetiology of bladder perforation remains uncertain. In the 90 paediatric perforations reported in the literature since 1977, 78 (87%) occurred in patients with a neurogenic bladder [44]. Eighty-seven per cent occurred in patients on CIC, with failure to catheterise documented in almost 20%. These patients with poor sensation and competent bladder necks are at high risk for developing asymptomatic over-distension of the augmented bladder.

Data concerning the risk for rupture in each type of augmentation are conflicting. It has been reported in all enteric segments, with an incidence of 5–7% reported in the largest series and so all must be considered to be at risk. Approximately half of the perforation cases in the literature were surgically explored. Of these cases, 72% demonstrated rupture through the bowel segment while the remainder ruptured through the anastomotic zone. Rupture within the first 4 months is at an anastomotic site in 80% [43].

Children with bladder perforation present with a variety of signs and symptoms ranging from silent urinoma to florid sepsis and shock [43]. Abdominal pain or radiating shoulder pain are common secondary to peritoneal irritation but may be absent in the myelomeningocoele patients with decreased abdominal sensation. Silent or painless presentation may be caused by loculation of the leak and may explain why some patients have been managed successfully with percutaneous drainage only. The cystogram has been the most commonly used diagnostic tool for perforation but has a 20% false negative rate [44]. A high index of suspicion for perforation in any augmentation patient should be maintained and immediate surgical exploration initiated in gravely ill patients. Delay in diagnosis and failure to adequately resuscitate the patient can lead to a rapid downhill course and death [43].

Neoplastic Progression

Interest in neoplasia in urinary reservoirs was stimulated by the high incidence found in patients with uretero-sigmoidostomies (see Chapter 11). In that human model and supported by animal studies, four components were necessary to maximise risk: an anastomosis between, and therefore the presence of, intestine and transitional urothelium, urine and stool. Together, these gave rise to an anastomotic cancer. In the case of a clam cystoplasty, three of these are present. In addition, both the bowel segment and the native bladder may have a malignant potential which is increased by the presence of urine. It is not surprising therefore to find in a 1996 literature review that 13 of the 16 cases (80%) were anastomotic [45].

A range of other malignancies has been reported both in the bladder and intestinal segments. In many of the reports up to 1996 the augmentation had been carried out for chronic inflammatory conditions such as tuberculosis and bilharzia. It is not possible to give a specific risk for patients with an augmentation, least of all for any particular bowel segment. Extrapolation from data on all types of reservoirs suggests that it is only marginally increased from normal.

From the clinical point of view it must be remembered that cancer can occur with a clam cystoplasty and it may be at a younger age than normal. Screening with regular cystoscopy or examination of urine cytology has not been successful, with most tumours found in the screening intervals. These are rapidly progressive and often fatal. The best defence is for patients, their families and their doctors to respond rapidly and appropriately to the standard symptoms of urological cancer and to any other suspicious change in reservoir behaviour.

Unique Complications of Gastrocystoplasty

Hypochloraemic Metabolic Alkalosis

Stomach mucosal segments placed into the urinary tract retain the ability to secrete hydrogen ions. The parietal cells responsible for hydrochloric acid secretion are found in the body and fundus of the bladder and are always present in the traditional gastric augmentation wedge. Metabolic abnormality after gastrocystoplasty occurs less frequently than after augmentation with bowel segments. However, several authors have reported severe hyponatraemic hypochloraemic metabolic alkalosis after gastrocystoplasty including Ganesan *et al.* [46] who reported it in 9 of 73 patients (12%) with one patient requiring take-down of the gastric segment.

Excess systemic bicarbonate is typically excreted by the kidneys into urine and theoretically neutralises acidic urine. Early reports of metabolic complications after gastrocystoplasty occurred in renal failure patients, leading to speculation that impaired renal excretion of bicarbonate was the cause of metabolic alkalosis [47]. Subsequent series have described serious post-gastrocystoplasty metabolic alkalosis in patients with normal renal function [48]. These patients experienced hyperchloraemia and hypocalcaemia secondary to vomiting and hydrochloric acid loss from the stomach flap. With potassium depletion, renal bicarbonate reabsorption can be increased, perpetuating the alkalosis that began with acid loss.

Hypergastrinaemia

Several authors have reported hypergastrinaemia in patients with metabolic alkalosis. In the in situ stomach, distension and increased intraluminal pH stimulate gastrin secretion from the antral G cells. Hydrochloric acid is then secreted by parietal cells in response to circulating gastrin. Augmentation using the antrum of the stomach might then be expected to result in increased acid secretion into the urine with bladder distension. The experimental and clinical data are conflicting. Tiffany *et al.* [49] described severe hypergastrinaemia after antral gastrocystoplasty in dogs. However, Lim *et al.* [50] reported 13 children with an antral gastrocystoplasty and normal gastrin levels. If incomplete denervation of the stomach flap occurs with mobilisation then, theoretically, retained G cells in the augmentation flap would secrete gastrin in response to bladder stretch. Retained antrum in the gastrocystoplasty wedge is usually avoided when the gastrocystoplasty wedge popularised by Adams *et al.* [51] is used as it avoids the lesser curve of the stomach. However, variable distribution of G cells is possible and selection of the wedge is sometimes more dependent on the distribution of vessels feeding the flap than the exact location on the stomach.

Again, there are conflicting data regarding the role of gastrin in post-gastrocystoplasty aciduria when the augmentation flap is harvested from the body of the stomach. Muraishi *et al.* [52] found elevated serum gastrin levels 3 months after gastrocystoplasty in dogs, but no persistence of hypergastrinaemia. These animals did develop mucosal erosions and ulceration in the augmented native bladder but no similar changes in the gastric mucosa. In a prospective study of gastrocystoplasties from the body of the stomach, Bogaert *et al.* [53] investigated gastrin secretion in response to bladder and stomach distension. They found an increase in serum gastrin after stomach distension with food, but no increase in acid secretion or serum gastrin with bladder distension. Urinary pH fell and titratable acids increased in parallel to serum gastrin increase. These data support the theory that gastrin secretion from in situ stomach acts on gastrocystoplasty parietal cells to produce acid.

Haematuria-Dysuria Syndrome

Haematuria-dysuria syndrome is a complication unique to bladder augmentation with full thickness stomach flaps. Strictly, it is defined as dysuria and haematuria (in the absence of infection), skin irritation or excoriation and suprapubic or perineal pain. Typically, the symptoms are mild and do not require medication, but the problem can be severe enough to require take-down of the gastric segment [47].

Since these early reports several authors have speculated on the possible aetiology of the syndrome. The reports are conflicting concerning the presence of aciduria. Dykes and Ransley [54] reported gross haematuria and severe dysuria after gastrocystoplasty in two of eight children with compromised renal function. One of these patients demonstrated normal serum chloride and gastrin levels, but elevated levels of urinary titratable acids. Both patients improved with oral omeprazole or H_2-receptor blockers. In the large series reported by Nguyen *et al.* [55] there was no difference between the pre-prandial and postprandial urine pH levels. Plawker *et al.* [48] found refractory metabolic alkalosis associated with haematuria and dysuria in one patient with renal insufficiency. This patient had severe hypergastrinaemia but, interestingly, alkaline urine. However, intravesical pH can be significantly lower than the pH of voided urine and this may account for the difference in findings reported by the various authors [55].

Other factors leading to the syndrome have been suggested. One case of haematuria-dysuria syndrome resolved after the child was started on intermittent catheterisation, suggesting that Valsalva voiding and incomplete emptying may exacerbate the problem [54].

Oliguria could be expected to exacerbate any irritative process just from the long exposure of the mucosa to urine between infrequent voids. In their original series, Nguyen *et al.* [55] found that symptoms occurred more frequently in patients with renal insufficiency. Similarly, Sheldon *et al.* [56] reported haematuria-dysuria in a patient with end-stage renal failure which resolved with transplantation. Urinary incontinence is a risk factor occurring in up to 60% of patients with the syndrome [55]. The child with a sensate perineum who dribbles urine is logically at higher risk for dysuria than the continent child or the child with decreased sensation.

Changes Over Time

The adverse changes over time are the development of stones, metabolic acidosis perforation and cancer; and the new bladder segment may contract, or develop a perforation at the junction of the bladder and bowel. Most of these matters are dealt with earlier in the chapter.

Adverse outcomes can occur for the upper renal tracts because of increased bladder pressure, because of failure of the augmentation procedure, or from obstruction or leaking from the surgery of either the bladder or upper renal tracts. In particular, obstruction can occur when both kidneys are preserved during a uretero-cystoplasty. Monitoring the renal status with an annual US and blood tests is an appropriate approach. New hydronephrosis, unchanged on reservoir emptying, is usually the first sign of obstruction. Further investigation with a MAG3 renogram is used to confirm functional obstruction. However, further anatomical data require cross-sectional imaging. MRI is currently the modality of choice but its use has to be weighed against the need for general anaesthetic in the young child.

The beneficial changes of augmentation include the continence that is achieved with the larger lower pressure bladder, which can improve over time. This improvement is because of the secondary favourable change in the native bladder that comes from the reduced detrusor work hypertrophy because the muscle is not contracting against a high resistance. Video-urodynamic studies of a uretero-cystoplasty show the effect best; namely, the patch expands as the native bladder contracts, with little change in intravesical pressure.

Perhaps the most important thing to tell girls as they grow up with an intestinal reservoir is that their urine will give a false positive human chorionic gonadotrophin antibody test for pregnancy (blue line test) on nearly 60% of occasions (see Chapter 11).

References

1 Tasker JH. Ileo-cystoplasty: a new technique: an experimental study with report of a case. *Br J Urol.* 1953; 25: 349–357.

2 Pike JG, Berardinucci G, Hamburger B, *et al.* The surgical management of urinary incontinence in myelodysplastic children. *J Pediatr Surg.* 1991; 26: 466–471.

3 Gilchrist RK, Merricks JW, Hamlin HH, *et al.* Construction of a substitute bladder and urethra. *Surg Gynecol Obstet.* 1950; 90: 752–760.

4 Gil-Vernet JM. The ileocolic segment in urologic surgery. *J Urol.* 1965; 94: 418–426.

5 Couvelaire R. La 'petite vessie' des tuberculeaux genito-urinaires: essai de classification place et variantes des cysto-intestino-plasties. *J d'Urol*, 1950; 56: 641.

6 Zinman L, Libertino JA. Technique of augmentation cecocystoplasty. *Surg Clin North Am.* 1980; 60: 703–710.

7 Winter CC, Goodwin WE. Results of sigmoidocystoplasty. *J Urol.* 1958; 80: 467–472.

8 Beseghi U, Casolari E, Del Rossi C, *et al.* Enterocystoplasty with a sigmoid patch in children with neurogenic bladder dysfunction. *Pediatr Surg Int.* 1994: 9: 82–85.

9 Dounis A, Gow JG. Bladder augmentation: a long-term review. *Br J Urol.* 1979; 51: 264–268.

10 Hasan ST, Marshall C, Robson WA, *et al.* Clinical outcome and quality of life following enterocystoplasty for idiopathic detrusor instability and neurogenic bladder dysfunction. *Br J Urol.* 1995; 76: 551–557.

11 Lapides J, Diokno AC, Lowe BS, *et al.* Followup on unsterile intermittent self-catheterization. *J Urol.* 1974; 111: 184–187.

12 Mitrofanoff P. Cystostomie continente trans-appendiculaire dans le traitement des vessies neurologiques. *Chir Pediatr.* 1980; 21: 297–305.

13 Woodhouse CRJ, Macneily AE. The Mitrofanoff principle: expanding upon a versatile technique. *Br J Urol.* 1994; 74, 447–453.

14 Politano VA, Small MP, Harper JM, *et al.* Periurethral teflon injection for urinary incontinence. *J Urol.* 1974; 111: 180–183.

15 Caione P, Lais A, De Gennaro M, *et al.* Glutaralgehyde cross-linked bovine collagen in exstrophy/epispadias complex. *J Urol.* 1993; 150: 631–633.

16 Montague DK. The artificial urinary sphincter (AS 800): experience in 166 consecutive patients. *J Urol.* 1992; 147: 380–382.

17 Buson H, Diaz DC, Manivel JC, *et al.* The development of tumors in experimental gastroenterocystoplasty. *J Urol.* 1993; 150: 730–733.

18 Klee LW, Hoover DM, Mitchell ME, *et al.* Long term effects of gastrocystoplasty in rats. *J Urol.* 1990; 144: 1283–1287.

19 Ortiz V, Goldenberg S. Hypergastrinemia following gastrocystoplasty in rats. *Urol Res.* 1995; 23: 361–363.

20 Reinberg Y, Manivel JC, Froemming C, *et al.* Perforation of the gastric segment of an augmented bladder secondary to peptic ulcer disease. *J Urol.* 1992; 148: 369–371.

21 Sumfest JM, Mitchell ME. Gastrocystoplasty in children. *Eur Urol.* 1994; 25: 89–93.

22 Di Benedetto V, Beseghi U, Bagnara V, *et al.* The use of gastrocystoplasty in patients with bladder exstrophy. *Pediatr Surg Int.* 1996; 11: 252–255.

23 Gosalbez R, Woodard JR, Broecker BH, *et al.* The use of stomach in pediatric urinary reconstruction. *J Urol.* 1993; 150: 438–440.

24 Shoemaker WC. Reversed seromuscular grafts in urinary tract reconstruction. *J Urol.* 1955; 74: 453–475.

25 Stothers L, Johnson H, Arnold W, *et al.* Bladder auto augmentation by vesicomyotomy in the pediatric neurogenic bladder. *Urology,* 1994; 44: 110–113.

26 Dewan PA, Owen AJ, Stefanek W, *et al.* Late follow-up of auto-augmentation omentocystoplasty in a sheep model. *Aust N Z J Surg.* 1995; 65: 596–599.

27 Dewan PA, Stefanek W, Lorenz C, *et al.* Auto augmentation omentocystoplasty in a sheep model. *Urology,* 1994; 43: 888–891.

28 Stohrer M, Kramer A, Goepel M, *et al.* Bladder auto-augmentation: an alternative for enterocystoplasty. *Neurourol Urodynam.* 1995; 14: 11–23.

29 Dewan PA, Byard RW. Auto-augmentation gastrocystoplasty in a sheep model. *Br J Urol.* 1993; 72: 56–59.

30 Dewan PA, Stefanek W. Autoaugmentation gastrocystoplasty: early clinical results. *Br. J.Urol.,* 1994 74:460–464.

31 Dewan PA, Stefanek W. Auto-augmentation colocystoplasty. *Pediatr Surg Int.* 1994; 9: 526–528.

32 Dewan PA, Condron SK. Extraperitoneal ureterocystoplasty with transuretero-ureterostomy. *Urology,* 1999; 53: 634–636.

33 McDougal WS. Metabolic complication of urinary intestinal diversion. *J Urol.* 1992; 147: 1199–1208.

34 Kass EJ, Koff SA. Bladder augmentation in the pediatric neuropathic bladder. *J Urol.* 1983; 129: 552–555.

35 Mitchell ME, Piser JA. Intestinocystoplasty and total bladder replacement in children and young adults: follow-up in 129 cases. *J Urol.* 1987; 138: 579–584.

36 Nurse DE, Mundy AR. Metabolic complications of cystoplasty. *Br J Urol.* 1989; 63: 165–170.

37 Hansson HA, Kock NG, Norlen L, *et al.* Morphologic observations in pedicled ileal grafts used for construction of continent reservoirs for urine. *Scand J Urol Nephrol.* 1978; 49(suppl.): 49.

38 Blyth B, Ewalt DH, Duckett JW, Snyder HM III,. Lithogenic properties of enterocystoplasty. *J Urol.* 1992; 148: 575–577.

39 Smith RB, Van Cangh P, Skinner DG, *et al.* Augmentation enterocystoplasty: a critical review. *J Urol.* 1977; 118: 35–39.

40 Hendren WH, Hendren RB. Bladder augmentation: experience with 129 children and young adults. *J Urol.* 1990; 144: 445–453.

41 Palmer LS, Franco I, Kogen SJ, *et al.* Urolithiasis in children following augmentation cystoplasty. *J Urol.* 1993; 150: 726–729.

42 Garzotto MG, Walker RD 3rd., Uric acid stone and gastric bladder augmentation. *J Urol.* 1995; 153: 1976.

43 Bauer SB, Hendren WH, Kozakewich H, *et al.* Perforation of the augmented bladder. *J Urol.* 1992; 148: 699–703.

44 Mansson W, Bakke A, Bergman B, *et al.* Perforation of continent urinary reservoirs: Scandinavian experience. *Scand J Urol Nephrol.* 1997; 31(6): 529–532.

45 Fernandez-Arjona M, Herrero L, Romero J, *et al.* Synchronous signet ring cell carcinoma and squamous cell carcinoma arising in an augmented ileo cystoplasty: case report and review of the literature. *Eur Urol.* 1996; 29: 125–128.

46 Ganesan GS, Mitchell ME, Nguyen DH, *et al.* Bladder reconstruction using stomach: 73 patients and 6 years later. *J Urol.* 1992; 147: 253A.

47 Kinahan TJ, Khoury AE, McLorie GA, *et al.* Omeprazol in post-gastrocystoplasty metabolic alkalosis and aciduria. *J Urol.* 1992; 147: 435–437.

48 Plawker MC, Rabinowitz SS, Etwaru DJ, *et al.* Hypergastrinemia, dysuria-hematuria and metabolic acidosis: complications associated with gastrocystoplasty. *J Urol.* 1995; 154: 546–549.

49 Tiffany P, Vaughan ED Jr, Marion D, *et al.* Hypergastrinemia following antral gastrocystoplasty. *J Urol.* 1986; 136: 692–695.

50 Lim STK, Lam SK, Lee NW, *et al.* Effects of gastrocystoplasty on serum gastrin levels and gastric acid secretion. *Br J Urol.* 1983; 70: 275–277.

51 Adams MC, Mitchell ME, Rink RC. Gastrocystoplasty: an alternative solution to the problem of urological reconstruction in the severely compromised patient. *J Urol.* 1988; 140: 1152–1156.

52 Muraishi O, Ikado S, Yamashita T, *et al.* Gastrocystoplasty in dogs: an ulcerating effect of acid urine. *J Urol.* 1992; 147, 242–245.

53 Bogaert GA, Mevorach RA, Kim J, *et al.* The physiology of gastrocystoplasty: once a stomach, always a stomach. *J Urol.* 1995; 153: 1977–1980.

54 Dykes EH, Ransley PG. Gastrocystoplasty in children. *Br J Urol.* 1992; 69: 91–95.

55 Nguyen DH, Bain MA, Salmonson KL, *et al.* The syndrome of dysuria and hematuria in pediatric urinary reconstruction with stomach. *J Urol.* 1993; 150: 707–709.

56 Sheldon C, Gilbert A, Wacksman J. Gastrocystoplasty: technical and metabolic characteristics of the most versatile childhood bladder augmentation modality. *J Pediatr Surg.* 1995; 30: 283–287.

10

Radiology and Follow-up of the Neobladder

Richard Hautmann and Bjoern G. Volkmer

Introduction

With improvements over the past several decades in surgical techniques, the morbidity associated with radical cystectomy (RC) has dramatically decreased. This has encouraged the development of a variety of techniques for bladder replacement. Construction of an intestinal reservoir with anastomosis to membranous urethra (orthotopic neobladder) is now standard in many institutions.

The Procedure

Radical Cystectomy in Females (Figure 10.1)

We prefer to spare the anterior vaginal wall if an orthotopic bladder substitute (OBS) is planned. This eliminates the need for vaginal reconstruction, helps to maintain the complex musculo-fascial support system and to prevent injury to the innervation of sphincter and proximal urethra, both important components of the continence mechanism [1]. There is an increasing tendency to preserve the uterus if oncologically safe. Oophorectomy is carried out in postmenopausal women.

Radical Cystectomy in Males (Figure 10.2)

RC is begun with an intra-fascial radical prostatectomy, in a retrograde fashion. At the base of the prostate, a 2–3-cm transverse incision of Denonvilliers' fascia is carried out, and vasa are transected preserving the seminal vesicles. A cleavage plane is easily developed anterior to the ampullae and seminal vesicles and dorsal to the trigone. The ascending cleavage plane reaches the cul-de-sac, with the inferior bladder pedicles still intact.

The remainder of the RC can be carried out in an ascending or descending fashion [2].

Following those modified RC techniques in both sexes, the pelvic floor anatomy resembles the original pre-operative situation most closely and provides the basis for successful orthotopic reconstruction and imaging.

The Neobladder

In 1987, the ileal neobladder was introduced by Hautmann *et al.* and the urethral Kock pouch by Ghoneim, and in 1988 the ileal bladder substitute by Studer *et al.* [3–5]. They were all made from ileum, detubularised and cross-folded and had anti-reflux protection by a Le Duc technique, a nipple and a 'triple nipple', respectively. In forming the reservoir, a 'chimney' of ileum is preserved either unilaterally or bilaterally for the anastomosis to the ureters (Figure 10.3).

Neobladders can also be made with large bowel but the outcomes are probably less satisfactory. The intraluminal pressure is

Radiology and Follow-up of Urologic Surgery, First Edition. Edited by Christopher Woodhouse and Alex Kirkham.
© 2018 John Wiley & Sons Ltd. Published 2018 by John Wiley & Sons Ltd.

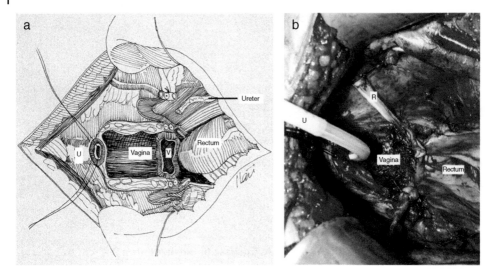

Figure 10.1 (a) Diagram of the final result of a precise modified anterior exenteration in a female with maximum preservation of the urethral support structures, the bottom of this defect being the anterior vaginal wall. U, urethra; V, open vaginal vault after removal of uterus. Note the considerably modified radicality as compared with standard radical cystectomy. (b) Operative photograph of the female pelvis (different patient). R, round ligament; U, urethra with catheter. Note the minimum excision defect following radical cystectomy with maximum preservation of support structures and nerves.

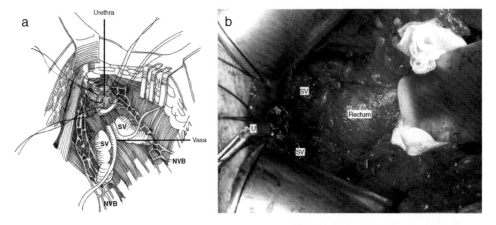

Figure 10.2 (a) Diagram of the final situation after seminal vesical sparing radical cystectomy. The seminal vesicles (SV) are preserved with neurovascular bundles (NVB) lateral and partly covered by them. (b) Corresponding operative photograph of the male pelvis. SV, seminal vesicles; U, urethra with a catheter.

higher and some spontaneous contractions persist so that continence is more difficult to achieve. The ureters are usually tunnelled into the colonic wall and there is no chimney.

Postoperative Imaging

In the immediate postoperative period, a cystogram is carried out at around 10 days to look for an anastomotic leak (Figure 10.4).

Figure 10.3 (a) Diagrams to compare the changes in radius (r), volume (mL) and pressure in insolated 40 and 60 cm bowel segments after detubularisation and cross-folding [12]. Note the lower volume and higher pressure found with only a single fold. The volume of a sphere is given by the formula $v = 4/3\pi r^3$ so that a small increase in radius gives a large increase in volume. *Source:* Simon *et al.* 2006 [12]. Reproduced with permission of Elsevier. (b) Diagrams comparing the same data in reservoirs constructed intracorporeally.

a

Principles of Open Orthotopic Reconstruction

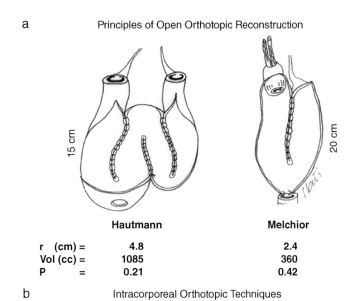

	Hautmann	Melchior
r (cm) =	4.8	2.4
Vol (cc) =	1085	360
P =	0.21	0.42

b

Intracorporeal Orthotopic Techniques

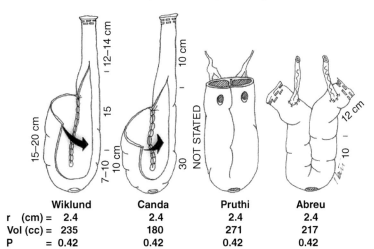

	Wiklund	Canda	Pruthi	Abreu
r (cm) =	2.4	2.4	2.4	2.4
Vol (cc) =	235	180	271	217
P =	0.42	0.42	0.42	0.42

In assessing later postoperative imaging it is essential to know which of the pelvic organs have been preserved. Similarly, the type of neobladder formation must be known. Typical 'normal' postoperative images are shown in Figures 10.5 and 10.6.

Long-term experience has shown that many functional and biochemical changes occur with the formation of an intestinal neobladder. Most are initially symptomless but prompt identification allows early management and sometimes prevents irreversible consequences (see also chapter 11).

Clinical Follow-up

The follow-up protocol that has been developed in Ulm is shown in Table 10.1.

Clinical Examination

Examination including the lymphatic and rectal systems is still a central part of

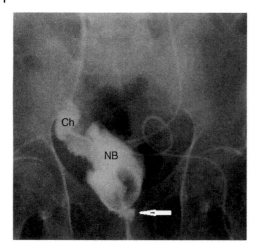

Figure 10.4 Cystogram of neobladder (NB) on day 10 postoperatively showing a small leak at the ileo-urethral anastomosis (arrowed). There is reflux into the chimney (Ch) and ureter on the right side. No left reflux into chimney or ureter. Stents are still in situ.

monitoring, especially for recurrent cancer. Development of hypertension can be an early sign of renal obstruction. For the urinary tract, where abnormalities are

seldom palpable, ultrasound (US) is an essential part of 'clinical' examination.

Bladder and Urine Investigations

Information on bladder control and emptying pattern are obviously required. New symptomatic infections, confirmed by stix testing and culture, are an early sign of the development of incomplete voiding. If the residual is more than 50 mL, the cause must be sought. Proteinuria is not a normal finding with intestinal reservoirs and should be investigated in the standard manner. Symptomless bacteriuria can be ignored.

Renal Investigations

Preservation of renal function is critical. Although the standard blood investigations are informative, the serum creatinine does not exceed laboratory norms until about 50% of glomerular function has been lost. A rising creatinine, even though within the normal range, is significant for renal deterioration. Such a finding, especially if combined with

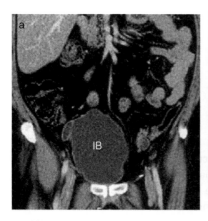

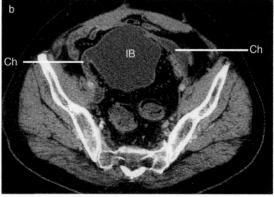

Figure 10.5 (a) Coronal CT to show an ileal neobladder (IB). The wall of the neobladder is uniformly thin. Note its position in relation to the pelvis – displacement from this position sometimes indicates local recurrence. (b) Transverse CT to show the neobladder. In this form of reconstruction there are two chimneys (Ch). (c,d,e) The chimneys are usually best seen on sagittal views. (c) A cystogram of an ileal neobladder taken about 10 days postoperatively to confirm absence of leaks. A, position of the anastomosis; C, chimney; U, ureter into which there is reflux . There is no leak. (d) A sagittal film from a CT scan at about 1 year post surgery. The chimney is marked with white arrows (note the narrowing from a peristaltic contraction). NB, neobladder. On transverse images such as (e), it is not possible to identify the chimney (arrowed C) without tracing down from the kidney or up from the bladder as it is indistinguishable from normal bowel. (f) Coronal T2-weighted MRI of a patient with an ileal neobladder (IB). For routine imaging of the urinary tract, MRI does not have any advantage over CT scan. The renal pelvises (K) are less well shown and the smooth thin neobladder wall is the same as on CT.

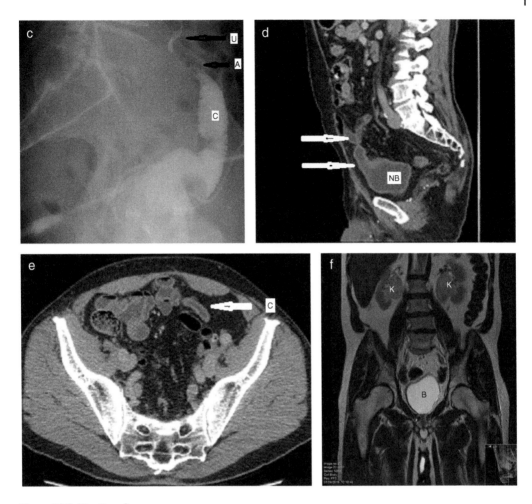

Figure 10.5 (Continued)

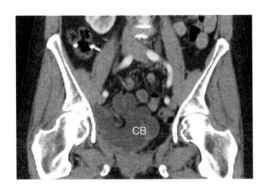

Figure 10.6 Coronal CT of a right colon neobladder (CB). Note that the wall is a little thicker than that of an ileal neobladder. The partially filled reservoir shows the irregular wall and wide-mouthed pouches.

hypertension and proteinuria, should trigger detailed nephrological investigation. Storage of urine in intestinal reservoirs is not, on its own, a cause of renal failure.

The age-related decrease in renal function is 9.1 mL/min/1.73 m^2 per decade after age 40 years in healthy patients. Functional deterioration is found in 30% and end-stage renal failure in 6.6% of patients after RC, irrespective of the type of urinary diversion [6].

There are two major factors following OBS that have a role in renal function deterioration.

1 *Obstruction* Obstruction of the lower ureter or uretero-intestinal anastomosis

Table 10.1 Follow-up schedule for patients with an ileal neobladder (Ulm experience).

Before surgery	After surgery	Months after surgery 3	6	12–15	18–21	24	30	36	42	48	54	60	Yearly
General													
×	Clinical examination	X	X	X	X	X	X	X	X	X	X	X	X
×	Body weight, blood pressure	X	X	X	X	X	X	X	X	X	X	X	X
×	US (if no CT/MRI)	X	X	X	X	X	X	X	X	X	X	X	X
×	Uroflow/residual urine	X	X	X	X	X	X	X	X	X	X	X	X
Blood tests													
×	Hb, creatinine, urea, Na, K, Mg, CI, Ca	X	X	X	X	X	X	X	X	X	X	X	X
×	Venous blood gas analysis/bicarb	X	X	X	X	X	X	X	X	X	X	X	X
	Folic acid, vitamin B_{12}					X		X		X		X	X
Urine tests													
×	Urine dip stick	X	X	X	X	X	X	X	X	X	X	X	X
×	Urine culture	X	X	X	X	X	X	X	X	X	X	X	X
×	Voiding diary	X	X	X	X	X	X	X	X	X	X	X	X
×	Voiding questionnaire	X	X	X	X		X	X		X			X
For patients with cancer													
×	Cytology (standard)		X	X	X	X	X	X	X	X	X	X	X
×	Alk phos, GOT, γ-GT	X	X	X	X	X		X		X		X	X
	Urethral washout cytology		X	X	X	X		X		X		X	X
	Forced diuresis for upper tract cytology		X		X		X		X		X	X	
×	CT thorax, abdomen, pelvis		X	X	X	X		X		X		X	
×	Bone scan		X	X	X	X						X	
	CT urogram (if upper tract history)			X		X		X				X	
Incidental prostate cancer													
×	PSA	X		X		X		X			X	X	

Alk phos, alkaline phosphatase; Ca, calcium; CI, chloride; CT, computerised tomography; γ-GT, gamma-glutamyltransferase; GOT, glutamic oxaloacetic transaminase; Hb, haemoglobin; K, potassium; Mg, magnesium; Na, sodium; PSA, prostate-specific antigen; US, ultrasound.

is a problem with all diversions or reconstructions. Early obstruction may be caused by oedema at the ureteric anastomosis which will usually resolve. Otherwise, obstruction may be a result of fibrous stenosis, ureteric kinking, tumour or stones (Figures 10.7 and 10.8).

When the right colon is used as a neobladder the ureters are anastomosed to the tail of the ileum so that the ileo-caecal valve prevents reflux. The valve is visible as an apparent filling defect and is a normal finding (Figure 10.9). The valve can occasionally act as an obstruction in which case both ureters will be dilated down to the ileo-caecal valve. Such obstructions can be corrected by a longitudinal valvotomy.

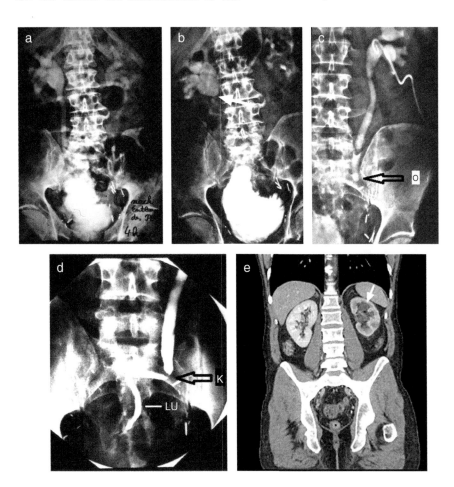

Figure 10.7 (a) A conventional intravenous urogram (IVU) at 4 hours showing delayed excretion on both sides. The patient was 6 weeks post cystectomy and maintaining reasonable renal function. (b) IVU of the same patient 2 months later showing good drainage on the left and a nearly empty right ureter. An underlying uretero-pelvic junction obstruction is shown on the right side (arrow). (c) Early film in an antegrade ureterogram series showing obstruction of the ureter at the level of the sacro-iliac joint (arrowed O). (d) A later film in the same antegrade series clarifies the situation of a kink (K) with some flow into the lower ureter (LU). (e) Coronal CT urogram showing delayed enhancement of the left kidney, some loss of parenchyma and hydrocalicosis (arrow) strongly suspicious of obstruction. (f) Antegrade ureterogram taken prone, of the same patient. There is complete obstruction (O). There is a faint filling defect at the obstruction which could indicate invasive tumour. (g) CT with contrast in the same patient, showing the presence of a stent (white) in the left ureter. The soft tissue around it, between the black arrows, is strongly suggestive of recurrent transitional cell carcinoma as the cause of obstruction. The diagnosis was confirmed on cytology washings from the ureter.

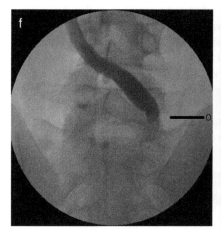
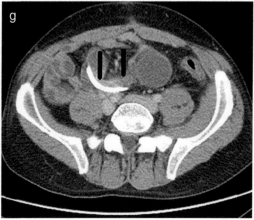

Figure 10.7 (*Continued*)

The great majority of stenoses occur within the first 1–2 years postoperatively, regardless of the type of ureteric anastomosis. However, the risk is still

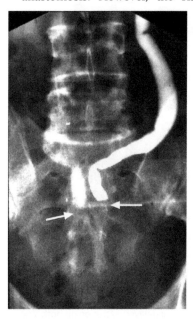

Figure 10.8 Bilateral antegrade ureterograms showing that both ureters are obstructed (arrows). This was because of local recurrence. Both ureters were anastomosed to the same chimney. A hazard of putting both ureters next to each other is that local recurrence is likely to affect both of them. This is true with all other diversions or reconstructions after cystectomy for transitional cell carcinoma of the bladder.

cumulative over time. Stenoses are often insidious and clinically silent. Flank pain and infection are usually a late manifestation except with stones. After cystectomy they are more commonly ischaemic, occurring after manipulation or radiation. Non-ischaemic strictures are normally caused by recurrent malignancy [6].

2 *Reflux* High pressure reflux of infected urine can cause renal function deterioration. However, the value of anti-reflux techniques in OBS is debatable. In four randomised trials there was no significant difference in serum creatinine, urine infection rates and bladder capacity between those with and those without an anti-refluxing anastomosis. A stricture was seen in 13.5% of patients with an anti-reflux nipple compared with 3% of patients with a refluxing technique [7].

Oncologic Follow-up Specific to the Neobladder

Local Recurrence

In our own series of 357 patients, local recurrence was diagnosed after evaluating pelvic symptoms with computerised tomography

Figure 10.9 CT of a colonic neobladder (arrowed NB) showing the ileo-caecal valve (arrowed ICV) which is characterised by an apparent filling defect in the neobladder but outlined by fat. This is a classic appearance of an ileo-caecal valve in any urinary reservoir.

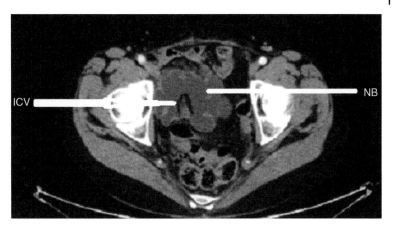

(CT) and US in 33 patients and incidentally in 10 who were asymptomatic during routine follow-up (12%). Pelvic and/or rectal pain was the most common presenting symptom (26 of 43 patients). Other clinical features that heralded the diagnosis included bowel obstruction in one patient, urinary retention in one, urethral bleeding in three, and inguinal and lower extremity oedema in two (Figure 10.10).

Median survival was 17 months and median time to recurrence was 10 months. Of the 43 patients with local recurrence at follow-up, 36 had had locally advanced cancer on the final pathological evaluation (stage pT3a or node positive, or worse). Seventeen of them had concomitant distant metastases. Of the 43 patients, 40 maintained good neobladder function until they died. Local recurrence interfered with the upper tract in 24 cases, neobladder in 10 and intestinal tract in 7. The neobladder was removed only in one patient because of a neovesical intestinal fistula [8].

Recurrence in the transitional urothelium may be in the upper tract (Figure 10.7f,g) or in the urethra. Out of 1420 neobladder patients, 25 cases of upper tract recurrence were observed. The overall rate at 5, 10 and 15 years was 2.4%, 3.9% and 4.9%, respectively. Upper tract recurrence did not develop in any patients with non-transitional cell carcinoma.

Four risk factors for upper tract recurrence were identified: history of carcinoma in situ or recurrent transitional cell carcinoma, cystectomy for non-muscle invasive cancer and tumour involvement of the distal ureter in the cystectomy specimen. Patients with transitional cell carcinoma who had none of these risk factors had an upper tract recurrence rate of only 0.8% at 15 years. The incidence rate increased with the number of positive risk factors, being. 8.4% in patients with one or two risk factors and 13.5% in those with three or four risk factors.

Patients who have undergone cystectomy for transitional cell carcinoma and with at least one risk factor for upper tract recurrence should have annual imaging of the kidneys and ureters.

Retrograde pyelography may be necessary if the patient is not a candidate for intravenous injection of contrast medium or if intravenous urography (normally with CT) is not diagnostic. Further evaluation of filling defects on imaging studies usually requires ureteroscopic evaluation. In practice, most upper tract recurrences are fatal with only about 27% surviving 5 years (Figures 10.7 and 10.8) [9].

The incidence of urethral recurrence after cystectomy is likely to be higher than that in the upper tracts as transitional cell carcinoma has a propensity to recur preferentially 'down stream' of the original. The figures

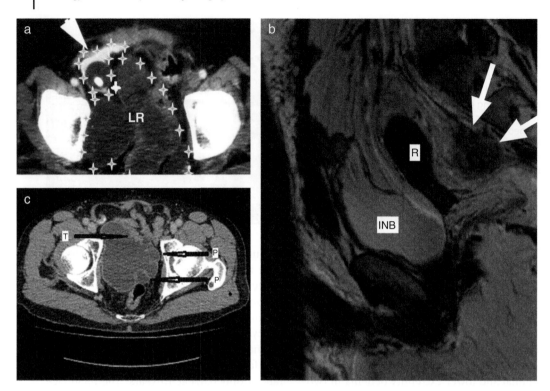

Figure 10.10 (a) Transverse CT to show a huge local recurrence (LR – yellow stars) of bladder cancer in the true pelvis. Despite gross displacement of the neobladder (arrow and green stars), function remained normal. The balloon of a Foley catheter (inserted for diagnostic purposes) can be seen in the neobladder. (b) When a smaller local pelvic recurrence of cancer is suspected, MRI may be useful, and has excellent soft tissue contrast resolution. In this case a T2-weighted sagittal image showing the relationship of the recurrence (arrowed) to the rectum (R) and neobladder (INB). In this case the bladder is not displaced (compare with a). (c) Axial enhanced CT image of a colonic neobladder. Not all filling defects in the neobladder are a result of recurrent tumour. Note that the wall is of less regular thickness; the area arrowed T is particularly thick. The outline is also irregular with multiple pouches (arrowed P). These are normal appearances and not signs of tumour recurrence or high pressure.

for incidence have wide variation from 1.4% to 18% at 5 years. There is dispute about predisposing factors, especially whether involvement of the prostatic urethra in the original tumour is relevant. It has been suggested that the incidence after neobladder formation is lower than that seen in a 'dry' urethra, although this may just reflect case selection. Cure of urethral recurrence depends on early diagnosis and lower grade. Urethroscopy is advocated annually and in response to urethral symptoms, especially bleeding [10, 11].

Secondary Tumour Growth in Urinary Diversions for Benign Disease (see also Chapter 11)

In 17 758 urinary diversions of all types, Kälble *et al.* [9] found 32 secondary tumours. The tumour risk in uretero-sigmoidostomy (2.58%) and cystoplasty (1.58%) was significantly higher than in other continent forms of diversion. The risk in (ileo-) colonic neobladders (1.29%) was significantly higher than in ileal neobladders. The difference

Table 10.2 Ninety-day complication rate in 1013 patients undergoing cystectomy and orthotopic neobladder formation at Ulm.

Complication	Percentage affected
Infections (various)	58
Genitourinary	17
Gastrointestinal	15
Wound related	9
Clavien 1 or 2	36
Clavien 3–5	22
90-day mortality	2.3

Source: Hautmann *et al.* 2013 [4]. Reproduced with permission of Elsevier.

between ileo-caecal pouches (0.14%) and ileal neobladders was not significant, and the tumour risk with ileal conduits was minimal (0.02%).

Uretero-sigmoidostomies, cystoplasties, and probably ileo-colonic neobladders, bear a significantly increased tumour risk compared with the general population and necessitate regular endoscopic evaluation from at least the fifth postoperative year.

Regular endoscopy is not useful after ileal neobladders and conduits. Imaging and endoscopic investigation are mandatory in the presence of symptoms such as hydronephrosis, chronic urinary infection or haematuria [7].

Complications

Complications up to 90 Days

Radical cystectomy and urinary diversion are two steps of one operation. However, the literature uniformly reports complications of the cystectomy while ignoring the fact that more than 75% of them are related to the diversion.

Of our 1013 orthotopic neobladder patients, 58% experienced at least one complication within 90 days of surgery, details of which are shown in Table 10.2 [7].

Long-term Complications

The long-term complication rate at Ulm was 40.8% (Table 10.3). As a result of the close routine follow-up many, especially

Table 10.3 Long-term (up to 20 years) complication rate in 1013 patients undergoing cystectomy and orthotopic neobladder formation at Ulm.

Complication		Percentage affected
Hydronephrosis		16.9
Incisional hernia		6.4
Febrile urinary infection		5.7
Ileus/small bowel obstruction		3.6
Outflow obstruction from neobladder	Tumour recurrence	1.1
	Anastomotic stricture	1.2
	Urethral stricture	0.9
Acidosis	Requiring bicarbonate therapy	33
	Severe metabolic acidosis	1
Chronic diarrhoea		0.8
Vitamin B_{12} deficiency		0.02

Source: Hautmann *et al.* 2013 [4]. Reproduced with permission of Elsevier.

those in the urinary tract, were found in a pre-symptomatic phase [7].

Changes Over Time

Reservoir Control

Incontinence

Continence of an orthotopic bladder reconstruction is undermined by two unavoidable consequences of radical cystectomy:

1 Loss of the afferent limb of the vesico-urethral reflex means that there is no coordination or functional relationship between reservoir and sphincter, as in a normal bladder;
2 Because of the loss of the spinal reflex activated by stretching of the muscle fibres of the native bladder, the sensation of normal desire to void is not felt.

In the daytime, the absence of reservoir–sphincter coordination is compensated for by activation of the urethro-sphincteric guarding reflex when there is reservoir over-filling or involuntary contractions. This guarding reflex could be estimated by measuring the maximum urethral closing pressure (MUCP) which reflects external sphincter activity. Diurnal continence is determined only by the condition of the external sphincter irrespective of the type of reservoir and whether it was constructed from a tubularised or a detubularised intestinal segment [13].

Nocturnal incontinence has been attributed to several causes, including loss of the vesico-urethral reflex, decreased muscle tone and urethral closure pressure during sleep, high amplitude involuntary contractions of the reservoir, decreased sensitivity of the membranous urethra and the shift of free water from the reservoir into concentrated urine.

Urodynamically, diurnal continence is determined by MUCP, while nocturnal continence is determined by the net result of two opposing forces that is MUCP vs. maximum contraction amplitude (Amp) plus baseline pressure at mid capacity (BAS). If MUCP is ≥47 cm H_2O, the patient should be continent during the day; if MUCP is ≥16 cm H_2O higher than the sum of Amp max and BAS mid, the patient would achieve continence during the night [13].

The reservoir control may deteriorate with time. Increasing age, use of colonic segments and non-nerve-sparing techniques have been suggested as risk factors for daytime urinary incontinence (UI) after OBS. Declining external urethral sphincter function, decreased sensory threshold in the membranous urethra and decreased vigilance of ageing patients are also possible explanations.

Voiding Failure (Hypercontinence)

Two types of OBS patients have been identified on the basis of voiding techniques:

1 Abdominal straining (Valsalva manoeuvre) used during the complete voiding episode.
2 Valsalva manoeuvre used only at the end of emptying.

Koraitim *et al.* [10, 11] have shown that the contribution of abdominal pressure to the driving force of urination varies in different types of orthotopic reservoir. Urine is evacuated mainly by abdominal straining in ileal neobladders, by contraction for sigmoid neobladders and by a more or less equal contribution of straining and contraction for ileo-caecal neobladders.

Over time, 4–8% of men and 30–50% of woman lose the ability to empty their reservoir (Figure 10.11). There are two main causes for emptying failure: subneovesical mechanical obstruction of the neobladder outlet and dysfunctional voiding. To define treatment options it is mandatory to determine the aetiology by radiological and invasive examinations.

Of the 655 men in our study, 11.5% had a least one episode of failure of emptying the neobladder requiring some form of therapy during follow-up. Failure was because of dysfunctional voiding in 3.5% and mechanical

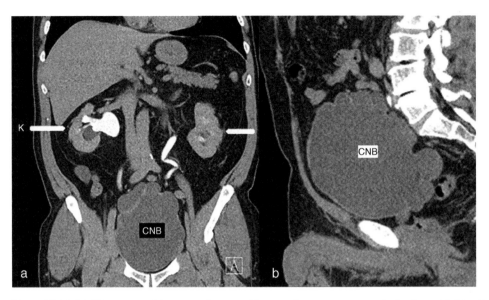

Figure 10.11 (a) CT urogram with contrast in a man 13 years after cystectomy and colonic neobladder. He has chronic retention with early dilatation of the upper tracts, especially on the right. Both kidneys show some scarring (kidneys arrowed and marked K). The colonic neobladder (CNB) is distended and many of the folds and diverticula normally seen with a colonic neobladder have been 'smoothed out' (compare with Figure 10.6). (b) A sagittal film of the CT showing the neobladder almost completely filling the pelvis.

obstruction in 8%. Causes of mechanical obstruction are shown in Table 10.3. In addition, non-urological malignancy (0.2%), 'mucosal valve' (0.5%) and a foreign body (0.2%) were implicated.

In 38 of 52 patients with mechanical obstruction of the neobladder, outlet emptying was fully restored with endo-urological procedures, while in 14 clean intermittent self-catheterization (CIC) was necessary. CIC was the therapy of choice for all patients with dysfunctional voiding.

Although the rate of transient or permanent neobladder emptying failure in males is high, most mechanical causes can be managed endoscopically [15].

The explanation for the much more common urinary retention in women (30–50%) has been more problematic. One theory has been the development of a posterior kink at the urethral anastomosis because of the loss of posterior support. Video-urodynamics and dynamic magnetic resonance imaging (MRI) studies seem to confirm the presence of a pouchocoele in women with high

residual urine and the absence of neobladder prolapse in those who void more completely.

There is an alternative theory that voiding dysfunction causing either retention or incontinence results from damage to autonomic nerves. Gross *et al.* [13] found that prior or concomitant hysterectomy and lack of attempted nerve sparing, shorter functional urethral length and lower MUCP were all associated with a higher risk of incontinence. They believed that retention was caused by either excess sympathetic tone resulting from denervation of the parasympathetic fibres or an atonic proximal urethra, presumably because of complete denervation, which collapsed on voiding to obstruct the outflow. The contribution of pre-operative urethral pressure profilometry needs to be confirmed in other prospective studies before it can be widely recommended [7, 16].

Other changes may be seen in future because of a failure to recognise the careful manner in which neobladder construction developed (Figure 10.3). The history of urinary diversion began in 1852 and started right away with continent diversion (i.e. uretero-sigmoidostomy) [17]. Anastomosing an intestinal reservoir to the urethra was proposed by Tizzoni and Foggi in 1888 [15].

After 25 years of successful OBS, recent developments ignore these basic principles. For instance, robotic reservoirs are constructed from short (40 cm) ileal segments, have significant non-detubularised sections and are only U-shaped (Figure 10.3). As a result, they have a small radius of 2.4 cm, geometric capacity of just 180–271 mL and pressure twice as high as a standard open OBS which has a radius of 4.8 cm and a geometric capacity as high as 1085 mL [19].

Day and night-time urinary incontinence has been reported in 7–13% and 14–43% of patients with an open OBS, respectively [19]. Regrettably, robotic series define continence, differently allowing diapers in 'continent' patients and report quality of life metrics instead of incontinence data. Using standard definitions, Canda *et al.* [20] reported as expected daytime continence in 65% of patients following robotic OBS but just 20% of the patients were dry at night. Thirty five per cent of all patients were totally incontinent; this included both the women in the series.

Metabolic Changes (see also Chapter 11)

Neurological defects caused by unrecognised vitamin B_{12} deficiency (optic atrophy, spinal cord degeneration, dementia and peripheral neuropathy) may be severe and irreversible. Patients should be monitored regularly for B_{12} deficiency following the use of ileum in a continent diversion [21].

Similarly, hyperchloraemic acidosis can develop at any time. With the monitoring described in Table 10.1, most cases will be identified when there are only small deviations of the serum bicarbonate and chloride from normal. At this point, supplementation with sodium bicarbonate should be started and the dose titrated until both parameters become normal.

References

1 Hautmann RE. The ileal neobladder. *Atlas Urol Clin North Am.* 2001; 9(2): 85–107.

2 Hautmann RE, Hautmann O, Volkmer BG, Hautmann S. Nerve-sparing radical cystectomy: a new technique. *Eur Urol (Suppl)* 2010; 9: 428–412.

3 Nassar OAH, Alsafa MES. Experience with ureteroenteric strictures after radical cystectomy and diversion: open surgical revision. *Urology.* 2011; 78(2): 459–465.

4 Hautmann RE, Abol-Enein H, Davidsson T, Gudjonsson S, Hautmann SH, Holm HV. ICUD-EAU international consultation on bladder cancer 2012: urinary diversion. *Eur Urol.* 2013; 63: 67–80.

5 Hautmann RE, Simon J. Ileal neobladder and local recurrence of bladder cancer: patterns of failure and impact on function in men. *J Urol.* 1999; 162: 1963–1966.

6 Volkmer BG, Schnoeller T, Kuefer R, Gust K, Finter F, Hautmann RE. Upper urinary tract recurrence after radical cystectomy for bladder cancer – who is at risk? *J Urol.* 2009; 182: 2632–2637.

7 Balci U, Dogantekin E, Ozer K, Gorgel SN, Girgin C, Dincel C. Patterns, risks and outcomes of urethral recurrence after radical cystectomy for urothelial cancer: over 20 year single center experience. *Int J Surg.* 2015; 13: 148–151.

8 Stein JP, Clark P, Miranda G, Cai J, Groshe S, Skinner DG. Urethral tumor recurrence following cystectomy and urinary diversion: clinical and pathological characteristics in 768 male patients. *J Urol.* 2005; 173(4): 1163–1168.

9 Kalble T, Hofmann I, Riedmiller H, Vergho D. Tumor growth in urinary

diversion: a multicenter analysis. *Eur Urol.* 2011; 60(5): 1081–1086.

10 Koraitim MM, Atta MA, Foda MK. Orthotopic bladder substitution in men revisited: identification of continence predictors. *J Urol.* 2006; 176: 2081–2084.

11 Koraitim MM, Atta MA, Foda MK. Desire to void and force of micturition in patients with intestinal neobladders. *J Urol.* 1996; 155: 1214–1216.

12 Simon J, Bartsch G Jr, Küfer JE, Gschwend BG, Volkmer BG, Hautmann RE. Neobladder emptying failure in males: incidence, etiology and therapeutic options. *J Urol.* 2006; 176: 1468–1472.

13 Gross T, Meierhans Ruf SD, Meissner C, Ochsner K, Studer UE. Orthotopic ileal bladder substitution in women: factors influencing urinary incontinence and hypercontinence. *Eur Urol.* 2015; 68: 664–671.

14 Simon M. Ectopia vesicae (absence of the anterior walls of the bladder and pubic abdominal parietes); operation for directing the orifices of the ureters into the rectum; temporary success subsequent death, autopsy. *Lancet.* 1852; 2: 568–570.

15 Tizzoni G, Foggi A. Die wiederherstellung der harnblase. *Zentralbl Chir.* 1888; 15: 921–924.

16 Hautmann RE, Egghart G, Frohneberg D, Miller K. The ileal neobladder. *Urologe A.* 1987; 26: 67–73.

17 Ghoneim MA, Kock NG, Lycke G, Shehab El-Din AB. An appliance free, sphincter-controlled bladder substitute: the urethral Kock pouch. *Urology.* 1987; 138: 1150–1154.

18 Studer UE, Casanova GA, Zingg EJ. Bladder substitution with an ileal low-pressure reservoir. *Eur Urol.* 1988; 141: 36–40.

19 Hautmann RE, Herr HW, Pruthi RS, Aron M. Robotic radical cystectomy – is the diversion the Achilles' heel? *J Urol.* 2014; 192: 1601–1603.

20 Canda AE, Atmaca AF, Altinova S, Akbulut Z, Balbay MD. Robot-assisted nerve-sparing radical cystectomy with bilateral extended pelvic lymph node dissection (PLND) and intracorporeal urinary diversion for bladder cancer: initial experience in 27 cases. *BJU Int.* 2012; 110(3): 434–444.

21 Matsui U, Topoll B, Miller K, Hautmann RE. Metabolic long-term follow-up of the ileal neobladder. *Eur Urol.* 1993; 24: 197–200.

11

General Consequences of Lower Urinary Tract Replacement and Reconstruction

Christopher Woodhouse and Alex Kirkham

Introduction

The lower urinary tract requires three components, which are largely independent of each other (Table 11.1): a reservoir in which to store the urine; a continence mechanism; and a conduit to conduct the urine to the surface. The reservoir can be constructed from any of the organs in the first column of Table 11.1, singly or in combination; the continence mechanism from the second; and the conduit from the third.

In general, reconstruction of the lower urinary tract with bowel has replaced incontinent diversion in children with congenital anomalies. In adults, the most common indication for reconstruction or diversion is cystectomy for cancer. Despite claims that orthotopic neobladder is the 'gold standard', there is no objective evidence that any one method is better than any other [1]. Although the various systems do not 'wear out', as some patients expect, they all have long-term problems which require surveillance. There are also complications caused by patient trauma and intercurrent events such as stone formation.

The consequences of intestinal reconstructions are brought about by three factors: the removal of the intestine from the gastrointestinal tract; the storage of urine within an intestinal reservoir; and the mechanical problems of the surgical reconstruction.

Reservoirs

The Stomach

The stomach, although it does have advantages, has not stood the test of time and now is only used if there is inadequate length of the other possible tissues and almost exclusively in children (see Chapter 9).

Ileum

Ileum has been the mainstay of reservoir construction. About 40 cm is needed to replace the bladder. Low pressure and a volume of 400–600 mL are achieved by longitudinal incision and re-formation in one of several possible formats. Lesser lengths of ileum are used to augment the bladder (clam cystoplasty). Sixty-five years of widespread use as some form of bladder substitute has given a good understanding of the long-term outcomes.

Gastrointestinal Consequences

Vitamin B_{12} Deficiency As vitamin B_{12} is absorbed from the terminal 15 cm of ileum, selection of a more proximal segment for bladder replacement or ileal conduit should allow normal absorption of the vitamin to continue. In practice this is not always the case. The body's store of B_{12} will last for about 4 years if absorption ceases completely. If there is reduced absorption, it may last for much longer. After exclusion of a long

Radiology and Follow-up of Urologic Surgery, First Edition. Edited by Christopher Woodhouse and Alex Kirkham.

Table 11.1 The components of the lower urinary tract and tissues available to replace it.

Reservoir	Continence mechanism	Conduit
Bladder	Urethral sphincters	Urethra
Stomach	Buried tube (e.g. Mitrofanoff)	Stomach tube
Ileum	Intussuscepted valve (e.g. Kock)	Ileal tube
Colon	Ileo-caecal valve	Appendix
Rectum	Artificial sphincter	Fallopian tube
Native urothelium	Anal sphincter	Anal canal
Artificial bladder		Ureter
		Skin tube
		Detrusor tube

segment of ileum from the gastrointestinal tract (GIT), there is a reduction in the level of B_{12} with time, especially beyond 7 years, even though it remains in the normal range. The actual length used does not seem to be a determining factor, but the mean B_{12} level of patients whose terminal 60 cm of ileum was spared is higher than those in whom it was partly incorporated in the urinary reservoir [2].

Vitamin B_{12} is involved in at least two protein synthesis pathways as a co-factor. Investigation of the pathways can be used to indicate early deficiency, before the B_{12} level itself becomes abnormal. For example, methyl malonic acid (MMA) accumulates in serum if there is inadequate B_{12} to metabolise it. In both children and adults, impaired B_{12} metabolism has been confirmed even when the absolute serum level is normal. Deficiency of B_{12} is found in about 21% of patients 7 years after creation of an ileal reservoir. More importantly, raised serum MMA may be found in a further 25% of patients [3].

Exclusion of the right colon, ileo-caecal valve and terminal ileum, as might be performed for a right colon reservoir, does not have the same consequences. Folic acid is absorbed from jejunum and so is not affected.

These findings presumably indicate that removal of ileum from the GIT reduces the absorption of B_{12}, so that late clinical deficiency will always remain a risk. Monitoring for low serum B_{12} is required from the fourth year after surgery and at least annually thereafter.

If the level is found to be close to the lower limit, a single injection of B_{12} should be given and the level re-measured at 3 months. Further supplements need only be given if the level falls close to the lower limit again. The deficiency is not the same as that encountered in pernicious anaemia when supplementation is required regularly and for life.

Other Malabsorption Consequences Nutritional deficiency is usually confined to children who have large sections of small bowel missing, as in cloacal exstrophy. In adults, the loss of 40 cm of terminal ileum trebles and of 100 cm increases fivefold the synthesis of bile acid. This predisposes to cholelithiasis, diarrhoea and steatorrhoea. A beneficial effect is a reduction in lipoproteins [4]. A biochemical marker of this is low serum carotene. In patients with a normal GIT and in an experimental study, the nutritional and functional consequences are not clinically significant [5].

Disturbances of defecation are a subject of some disagreement. In many series they are not mentioned at all or are said not to occur. There may be differences between patient groups or some clinicians do not specifically enquire about this. When specifically sought, disturbance of bowel function in otherwise uncomplicated patients is found in about 15% after ileal conduit or clam cystoplasty [6]. In patients having reconstruction after cystectomy for cancer, few have bowel disturbance and it is usually not bothersome.

An interesting group is those with idiopathic detrusor instability. Fifty-four per cent of patients report new bowel symptoms after ileal conduit or clam cystoplasty, including diarrhoea, incontinence and leakage of flatus. As a result, up to one-third regret having the operation [6]. When such symptoms occur, they do not improve with time, at least up to 8 years [7].

Storage Consequences

There may be an overlap between gastrointestinal and urine storage consequences. From the biochemical point of view, hyperchloraemic acidosis (HCA) is the most important (see Colon reservoirs). Because of the osmotic gradient, water may be lost into the reservoir through the ileal wall.

The most serious problems arise from the absorption of drugs and abnormal constituents excreted in urine. The cytotoxic drug methotrexate is one such. Although not commonly used now, it will cause severe bone marrow toxicity if forgotten. If it is administered, the reservoir should be drained with a catheter throughout treatment, blood levels checked and folinic acid rescue given.

An interesting problem arises with glucose in urine stored in ileum. If glucose is instilled into ileal conduits in non-diabetic patients, it is not absorbed. In insulin-dependent diabetic patients, it may be absorbed. This can cause hyperglycaemic ketoacidosis without measureable glycosuria. The experiment has not been repeated with ileal reservoirs but is unlikely to have a different result. As the ileal mucosa atrophies with time, the phenomenon may resolve with longer follow-up, but not always [8].

Colon

About 20 cm of colon is needed completely to replace the bladder. It is detubularised by longitudinal incision and re-formed in a 'U' shape. The pressures in right colon and, particularly the sigmoid colon, are higher than in ileal pouches.

Gastrointestinal Consequences

Colon has little metabolic activity. Its main function is to store the effluent from the ileum which may be up to 1.5 L/day. Ninety-nine per cent of this is absorbed as water. Some ions are exchanged and any carbohydrate remaining is converted to short chain fatty acids and absorbed. None of this produces a significant problem when 20 cm is excluded for urinary reconstruction except in those at risk of dehydration or faecal incontinence.

The distal colon forms and stores stool. Reduction in the length of colon, especially the sigmoid, may loosen the stools sufficiently to cause precipitancy or even incontinence.

Storage Consequences

Hyperchloraemic Acidosis Both ileal and colonic reservoirs can be responsible for HCA, but the more distal the colon used, the higher the incidence. There is some dispute about the mechanisms by which the serum bicarbonate becomes too low and the chloride too high. Much of the experimental work dates from more than 50 years ago.

When the urine has been mixed with faeces in the colon for even a short time, the slurry becomes very alkaline because of the high levels of bicarbonate and ammonia. At least in experimental animals the speed of development and the severity of the acidosis is proportional to the surface area of the colon in contact with urine [9].

The production of ammonia is by the action of urease producing faecal bacteria. Urinary urea is essential in making the slurry alkaline and producing the full syndrome. If urine is stored in an isolated rectum with no faeces present (as in the Boyce–Vest diversion) patients have hyperchloraemia but are not acidotic according to the plasma bicarbonate level [10].

In an experimental study where artificial urine was instilled into a variety of intestinal reservoirs, all patients were found to absorb sodium and potassium but the extent was variable. One-third of patients (but 50% of those with an ileo-caecal reservoir) were found to have hyperchloraemia. All had abnormal blood gases, the majority having metabolic acidosis with respiratory compensation. This was found even in patients with a small segment of bowel as in a clam cystoplasty. The findings were unrelated to renal function or to the time since the reservoir was constructed [11].

There is good evidence in humans that the normal response of the colon to the presence of an acid medium is secretion of bicarbonate and that this is the cause of the acidosis [12]. There are active transport mechanisms for the exchange of electrolytes throughout the intestine. Therefore HCA can occur with storage in any reservoir except the stomach. It is most common with a rectal reservoir (Table 11.2).

Although low plasma and total body potassium have been reported, they are not consistent findings. When allowance is made for uncorrected metabolic acidosis it is probable that normal total body potassium is maintained. Care must certainly be taken in prescribing potassium supplementation just on the basis of low plasma potassium [13]. If potassium is lost, it is not by exchange, but by the diarrhoea that can occur with

Table 11.2 Venous blood biochemical and haematological changes in patients with intestinal urinary reservoirs. Data are very unreliable and the incidences may be taken with a pinch of salt. The denominators are usually unknown, follow-up variable and definitions poorly described. The more the abnormalities are sought, the more often they are found. Arterial blood gas analyses give higher incidences for pH changes.

Reservoir	Biochemical/ haematological change	Incidence (%)
Stomach	*Hypo*chloraemic, metabolic alkalosis	0–24
Ileum	*Hyper*chloraemic metabolic acidosis	9–50
Ileum	Vitamin B_{12} deficiency	21+
Colon/rectum	*Hyper*chloraemic metabolic acidosis	50–100

uretero-sigmoidostomy or by the osmotic diuresis caused by excess urea reabsorbing from the colon [13, 14].

Fortunately, there is some ability to compensate for the bicarbonate loss. As the bicarbonate concentration in the colon becomes excessively high, diffusion occurs back into the bloodstream of the colon. Many patients thus stabilise in mild acidosis [12].

HCA is usually found from the routine annual blood test. We have not noted symptoms in any patient with biochemical HCA, even with bicarbonates as low as 15 mmol/L. Acute HCA is usually a consequence of an acute illness, particularly pyelonephritis. The presentation then is of that illness and the HCA is found on biochemical analysis. Even without an obvious associated illness, severe HCA is usually associated with hyperammonaemia which produces encephalopathy and coma.

The long-term consequences of HCA are uncertain. The older literature describes osteomalacia and vitamin-resistant rickets. All of the patients had severe and uncorrected HCA. They presented with bone pain, tenderness and weakness, but demineralisation must be far advanced before radiological changes are seen. This relationship has become less clear with time and contemporary reports on reconstruction have not detected osteomalacia or rickets [15].

In Wistar rats, there is a marked reduction in cancellous bone volume and strength after ileo-cystoplasty. There is even greater loss if the cystoplasty is accompanied by an additional resection of ileum. None of the animals were acidotic at sacrifice. If these findings could be transferred to humans, the implications are that the vertebrae, particularly, would be at increased risk of compression fracture and that the cause is not HCA. The increased effect of ileal resection with cystoplasty suggests that malabsorption from the ileum and absorption from the urine of unknown metabolites may be causative [15].

Clinical evidence is inconclusive. Minor degrees of HCA may produce osteomalacia [16]. In children, this would have a major impact on bone growth. In a small group of children, dual energy X-ray absorptiometry (DEXA) scanning showed a reduction in bone mineral density in the lumbar spine associated with HCA. This finding would be in keeping with the rat model [17]. In four of the six children for whom there were sufficient data, re-mineralisation occurred with correction of the HCA [18].

When osteomalacia does occur, it is not accompanied by hypercalciuria either clinically or experimentally [16]. Patients do not have nephro-calcinosis but renal stones occur as a relatively early complication in about 2% of patients surviving at least 6 months [19].

Although the long-term consequences of HCA are uncertain, there is enough evidence to treat it. Pragmatically, borderline HCA has been defined as an abnormality of either the serum bicarbonate or of the chloride. Definite HCA is an abnormality of both. Measurements must be made at least annually as HCA can occur at any time. Sodium bicarbonate 500 mg (6 mmol) twice daily is the starting dose and it is increased until both parameters come into the normal range. It is rare to find that treatment can be stopped, although the dose can sometimes be reduced.

Treatment of established osteomalacia is principally of the HCA with alkalis, reduced dietary chloride and supplementation of calcium and phosphorus. The role of vitamin D is unclear: patients have been shown to recover without supplementation but recovery is likely to be faster if it is given early in small doses such as 10 000–100 000 units of D_2 daily [20].

Rectum

The conventional uretero-sigmoidostomy stores urine at a pressure of about 40 cm H_2O [21]. The pressure rises as the rectum fills and the walls are less compliant than urologists are used to seeing in the bladder [22]. During sleep, although the rectal pressure falls so does the anal pressure, which increases the risk of nocturnal incontinence [21].

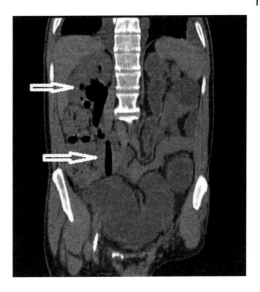

Figure 11.1 Coronal CT scan of a patient with a Mainz II variation of the uretero-sigmoidostomy showing gas in the renal pelvis, calyces and ureter (arrows).

The high rectal pressure increases the incidence of reflux into the kidneys, leading to infection (Figure 11.1). In some patients there is also reflux of urine up the colon as far as the caecum (Figure 11.2). As the severity of HCA is proportional to the surface area of bowel in contact with urine, patients have a biochemical problem that is difficult to control.

The success of the ileal conduit considerably reduced the use of the ureterosigmoidostomy. The realisation that the conduit was not as good as it originally appeared and the development of continent diversion eventually led to a small renaissance [23]. The important change was based on creating a low pressure reservoir by augmentation or re-forming of the rectosigmoid area [10].

The only system of low pressure rectosigmoid pouch that remains in use is the Mainz II. In this operation, the upper rectum and lower sigmoid are opened longitudinally over 20 cm and conformed into a 'U'-shaped reservoir. It has a mean pressure over 24 hours of 8.7 cm water, rising to 13.8 cm when full. The mean capacity is 520 mL (range 270–650 mL). There is no

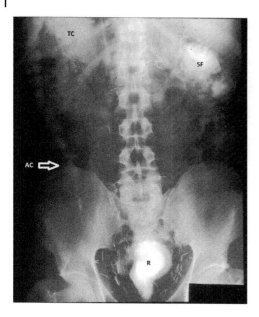

Figure 11.2 Delayed film of an intravenous urogram of a patient with a conventional uretero-sigmoidostomy showing contrast refluxing up the colon as far as the right side. AC, ascending colon; R, rectum; SF, splenic flexure; TC, transverse colon.

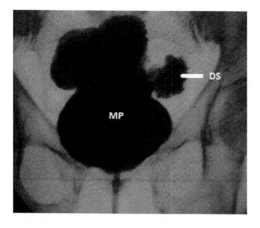

Figure 11.3 'Pouchogram' of a Mainz II recto-sigmoid pouch (MP) showing minimal reflux of contrast into the descending colon (arrow, DS).

reflux into the descending colon at these volumes (Figure 11.3) [24].

Continence (Mainz II)
The published continence rates are remarkably consistent at 92–100% by day and

marginally lower at night [25]. Investigation suggests that the main cause of incontinence is a deterioration of the anal sphincter pressure, particularly the maximum anal closing pressure (MACP), which is found in patients who are incontinent after surgery. On investigation pre-operatively, patients had a mean MACP of 232 mmHg compared to 194 mmHg postoperatively. However, in a retrospective portion of the investigation, incontinent patients had a MACP of 117 mmHg (SD $\pm$ 14) [26]. Assuming this to be the case, in addition to the traditional test of filling the rectum with 500 mL porridge to test continence, anal manometry could be used to identify patients with a MACP of <200 mmHg who would be predictably incontinent with a Mainz II. Incontinence is difficult to manage. The effluent is still foul smelling and only nappies will contain major leakage.

Very occasionally, there is a correctable problem in the rectosigmoid reservoir. The capacity can be measured by filling with X-ray contrast to see at what volume it refluxes into the descending colon. If it is less than about 350 mL, augmentation of the pouch with ileum may be helpful. Similarly, anorectal manometry may show a pouch with a higher pressure than the anal sphincter can control and augmentation may improve matters.

If it does become necessary to abandon a Mainz II diversion, the pouch should not be left in situ as it becomes a repository for inspissated faeces of ever-enlarging capacity. It may be possible to re-tubularise it or use it for urine storage. Otherwise it has to be removed.

In patients presenting with a conventional uretero-sigmoidostomy that has been continent for many years but has become incontinent, it is tempting to make a conversion to a Mainz II. In our own series, this was only successful in two of four patients. The acquired incontinence is more complicated and requires the help of a colorectal service. Unless there is an identifiable cause, a different diversion should be made [25].

Anastomotic Cancer

Much the most important consequence of diverting urine into the rectum is cancer at the anastomosis between the ureters and the bowel, first reported in 1929 [27].

Aetiology The tumours arise at the anastomosis or very close to it in more than 90% of cases (Figure 11.4). In patients diverted for benign disease, 95% are adenomatous but other types have been reported [28]. There has been some controversy on whether it is a tumour of the colon or of the ureter following adenomatous metaplasia. As tumours occur only at the anastomosis and not in adjacent areas, particularly not on the wall opposite the anastomosis, it seems best to consider the anastomosis as the primary site. This would also concur with the experimental findings in animals.

The most important aetiological factor both experimentally and clinically is the confluence of urine and faeces at the anastomosis between the urothelium and the colon.

In rats, the union of the urinary and faecal streams is as powerful a carcinogen as dimethylhydrazine (DMH) or N-[4-(5-nitro-2-furyl)-2-thiazoly] formanide (FANFT) which are very potent urinary and bowel carcinogens, respectively. Union of the urinary tract with the colon but with faeces excluded does not precipitate tumours [29]. In humans, the same applies: tumours occur when the two streams are mixed. They are rare in isolated colon conduits or reservoirs.

It must be remembered that the colon is a common site of adenocarcinoma and in patients under 40 years old 60% are in the sigmoid colon [30]. Cancer in intestine exposed to urine may be spontaneous and unrelated to the urinary diversion. In a literature review in 2004, five adenocarcinomas were identified in colon conduits and nine in colonic reservoirs [31]. Eight of these 14 occurred in less than 10 years from formation of the diversion and an indeterminate number were not at or even near the ureteric anastomosis. As the latency for the anastomotic tumour of the uretero-sigmoidostomy is at least 12 years, many of those in this review may have been colon primaries occurring, coincidentally, in the pouch (Figure 11.5a). Metastases may also occur in urinary reconstructions (Figure 11.5b). Anastomotic tumours are not seen if faeces are excluded.

The increased risk of carcinoma in patients with uretero-sigmoidostomy has been estimated at 1726 times that of the normal population [32].

In humans, the carcinogenic agent may be an N-nitroso compound produced from urinary nitrates and faecal secondary amines.

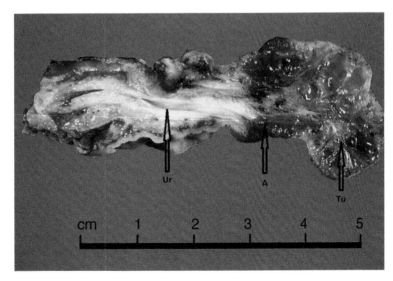

Figure 11.4 Fresh surgical specimen opened to show the relationship between the ureter (Ur), the anastomosis to the colon (A) and the tumour (Tu) which in this case was a benign adenoma.

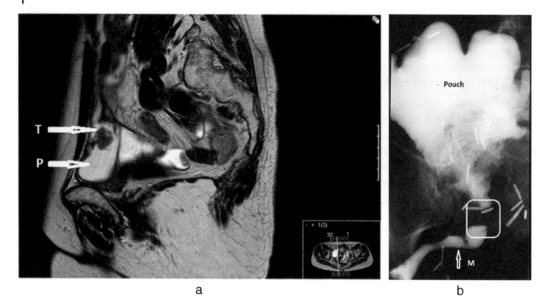

Figure 11.5 (a) A sagittal magnetic resonance image (MRI) of a carcinoma (arrow, T) in a right colon reservoir (arrow, P). This patient had multiple dysplastic polyps elsewhere in the colon and the tumour in the reservoir was assumed to be a carcinoma of the colon rather than a result of urine in a reservoir. (b) A pouchogram (Pouch) with an obstructed Mitrofanoff catheterisable conduit (arrow, M) due to a metastasis from a carcinoma of the cervix (outlined); the patient had previously had an anterior pelvic exenteration.

These potent carcinogens are present in uretero-sigmoid effluent in a concentration 10 times greater than in normal bladder urine. The concentrations in isolated colonic and ileal conduits are variable between patients. The only consistent finding is that it is lower when the urine is sterile [33].

The predisposing factor for neoplasia is that there has *ever* been an anastomosis between the urinary and faecal streams. Thus, the anastomosis is at risk in patients whose diversion has been changed from a uretero-sigmoidostomy to another system, leaving the ureteric anastomosis in situ.

Presentation and Management Now that the natural history of the condition is well understood, all cases should be found at screening sigmoidoscopy. However, patients presenting with 'haematuria' or anastomotic obstruction should be investigated with this diagnosis in mind. A normal ureteric orifice is shown in Figure 11.6(a) but some can look like tumours. On the other hand,

tumours as small as 8 mm may be malignant (Figure 11.6b).

The shortest recorded period of exposure to risk that resulted in an anastomotic cancer is 9 months. In other case reports, a benign neoplasm occurred after 2 years of exposure and the oldest malignancy for a patient diverted in childhood is 49 years.

The mean time from formation of the uretero-sigmoidostomy to the development of an anastomotic tumour is 18 years for a benign polyp and 25 years for a malignant adenocarcinoma. It is presumed that the 'benign' tumours become malignant over 5–10 years. Overall, the risk of any neoplasia is 22% at 20 years and about 30% at 30 years after the formation of uretero-sigmoidostomy [28, 34].

When found at annual screening flexible sigmoidoscopy, tumours should be in a pre-malignant state. They can then be treated by local excision of the anastomosis and a cuff of colon [35]. Although this renews the risk of neoplasia, it is the

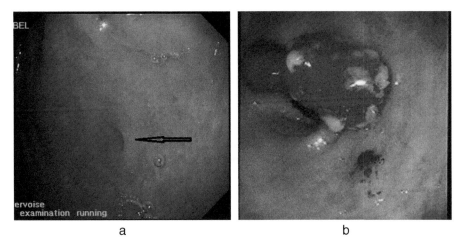

Figure 11.6 (a) Endoscopic view of a normal ureteric orifice in the colon (arrow). (b) An 8-mm anastomotic neoplasm that was malignant on histology. Source: Woodhouse 2015 [37]. Reproduced with permission of John Wiley and Sons.

choice of at least two-thirds of affected patients [36, 37].

No neoplasms have been reported in a modified uretero-sigmoidostomy, such as the Mainz II. However, it would be naive to think that there was no risk. Screening by appropriate endoscopy is required for the groups at risk.

Urodynamic Findings

Providing enough bowel is used, all segments can be made into a low pressure storage reservoir. At least in neobladder reservoirs in cystectomy patients, urodynamic compliance and pressure is better with ileum than with an ileo-colonic segment (see Chapter 10). For capacities, ileo-colonic segments are very similar to ileum alone [38]. Sigmoid colon reservoirs are one-third smaller than the others and a have a worse compliance (mean of 11 mL/cm water vs. 34 mL/cm water) [39].

Stones

Of the many problems that are a consequence of storing urine in an intestinal reservoir,

urolithiasis is one of the most common. Stones, especially in the reservoir, can occur in up to 53% of patients and have a high tendency to recur. The incidence increases gradually with length of follow-up; the mean time to stone formation is between 24 and 45 months (range 1 month to 10 years) [40]. The observation that some patients form stones repeatedly and others never do, even after 15–20 years of observation, suggests that there are factors other than just urine storage in bowel to be identified.

Most of the stones contain more calcium phosphate (CaP) than magnesium ammonium phosphate (MAP) and this is to be expected, as CaP is the first salt to crystallise out as urinary pH rises above 6; MAP generally crystallises out only at pH values above 7 and in the presence of a urinary tract infection with a urea-splitting organism. Some stones form in sterile urine (14% in our patients) and are usually a mixture of calcium oxalate and calcium phosphate [41]. The low pH in gastrocystoplasties protects them from stone formation and they are also rare in clam cystoplasties.

Urolithiasis is considered to be a multifactorial problem, including urinary stasis, infection, post-void residual (PVR) and foreign bodies [42, 43].

In patients with intestinal reservoirs, there are significant differences in urine composition and diet between stone formers and non-stone formers. Two-thirds of stone formers are either hypercalciuric (>6 mmol/day), all of whom have a renal leak of calcium because of a high intake and throughput of sodium, or have mild hyperoxaluria (>0.45 mmol/day).

In non-stone formers, the mean 24-h urine volume is 41% higher and the mean citrate excretion is 173% higher than in repeated stone formers. Urinary pH is 6.46 (range 6.0–7.0) in non-stone formers and 6.93 (range 6.3–7.8) in stone formers. Eighty per cent of stone formers have high risks for three or more types of stone [44]. The features protective against reservoir stone formation are shown in Table 11.3 [41].

The role of mucus is uncertain especially as neither patients nor doctors have an easy means of measuring it. Scanning electron microscopy and energy dispersive X-ray spectrometry show that the mucus of stone formers has increased calcium, phosphate, magnesium and calcium to phosphate ratio than that of non-stone formers [45]. When small stones are removed from a reservoir, there seems to be a spectrum of material from mucus through a chalk-like material to frank stone, suggesting that mucus might be a nidus for crystallisation (Figure 11.7). However, at least in children, neither clean intermittent catheterisation (CIC) nor mucus on their own are causative factors [46].

Those who void 'naturally' through the urethra seldom, if ever, form stones. There are conflicting results for patients who use CIC either through the urethra or through a Mitrofanoff channel at the top of the neobladder which suggests that there is little clinically significant difference [40, 46, 47].

Stone formation in intestinal reservoirs remains a common problem. Stones can grow very quickly. Large stones, as in Figure 11.8, are best removed by open surgery. Endoscopic removal, especially through a small catheterisable channel such as a Mitrofanoff, is difficult. The instruments have to be no bigger than 14 Fr. Even when stones are fragmented, the small particles adhere to the intestinal mucosa and are difficult to wash out. Stones of 1–2 cm can be removed percutaneously [48].

Table 11.3 Guidance on prevention of stones in intestinal urinary reservoirs. Based on theoretical data. There is no evidence that stone incidence is reduced with these regimes.

	Notes
Urine output >2 L/day	Equivalent to intake of 3–4 L/day or 4–6 L/day in hot weather
High fibre	Binds calcium in gut
Low oxalate	Spinach, beetroot, nuts, chocolate, soya beans, tea without milk
Moderate calcium (2–3 servings/day)	Serving = 1/3 pint milk, small yoghurt, 1 scoop ice cream
4–5 oz (140–160 g) animal protein/day	
5 servings fruit/day	
Low carbohydrate	
Low salt (especially 'junk food')	
No supplements of vitamins C or D	
Reservoir washout at least ×2/week	Might washout stone crystals before they form stones
Ensure complete reservoir emptying	
Empty reservoir at least 4-hourly	Longer intervals may increase UTI risk

UTI, urinary tract infection.
Source: Hamid *et al.* 2008 [41]. Reproduced with permission of John Wiley & Sons.

Figure 11.7 Clinical photograph showing a mixture of small stone fragments mixed with mucus and larger stones, removed from an intestinal reservoir. Source: Woodhouse 2015 [37]. Reproduced with permission of John Wiley and Sons.

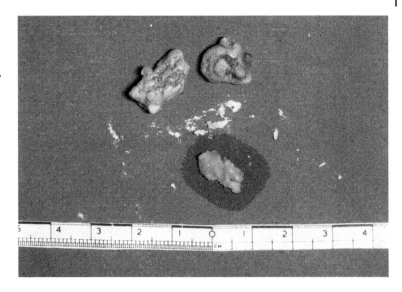

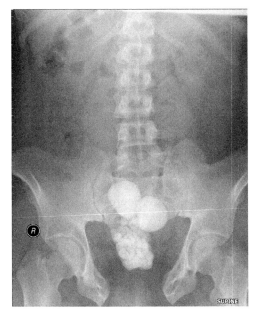

Figure 11.8 Plain X-ray in a boy born with exstrophy (note the open pelvic ring) to show two large and many small stones in a urinary reservoir.

Renal Function

A review of the literature from 2000 to 2013 concluded that the storage of urine in any intestinal reservoir does not, in itself, damage renal function [49]. Unfortunately, only 41 papers were evaluable, only three of which were controlled trials and the quality was generally poor. Most of the data apply to adults having cystectomy. Ureteric obstruction is much more damaging than reflux.

Part of the regular follow-up of patients with urinary diversions should include a measurement of renal function. As a routine, annual renal and reservoir ultrasound (US) and serum creatinine are sufficient. However, if either shows deterioration, a chromium ethylenediaminetetraacetic acid (EDTA) measurement of the glomerular filtration rate (GFR) should be performed. It is important to do the renal US with the reservoir both full and empty – apparent hydronephrosis often resolves when the reservoir is empty and this is a normal finding not indicative of renal damage (Figure 11.9).

If renal function is found to be deteriorating, the search should begin for an underlying cause. If there is a steady rise in creatinine over time, the most likely culprits are ureteric obstruction or consistent failure to empty efficiently. Step-like rises are more often a result of repeated episodes of pyelonephritis.

Perforation

Much the most dangerous complication of an intestinal reservoir is perforation. The

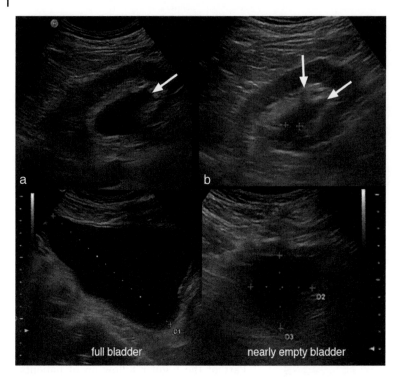

full bladder   nearly empty bladder

Figure 11.9 Ultrasound images of the right kidney in a patient with an ileal neobladder (a) before and (b) after bladder emptying (the corresponding bladder images are shown below). Note the degree of calyceal dilatation (arrows) is markedly less after bladder emptying.

peritoneal cavity becomes contaminated with urine which is likely to be infected. Patients develop peritonitis. In many cases there is rapid deterioration with septic shock over 24–48 hours. If not treated effectively it will be fatal.

The incidence is about 2% in colon reservoirs and about 1.3% in ileal ones at a mean follow-up of 22 months [50]. The risk does not disappear with time and longer follow-up produces more cases, with an incidence of 4.5–5% beyond 10 years [51]. Most perforations occur with a full reservoir, especially in the mornings and sometimes after minor trauma (including catheterisation). Young age and spina bifida strongly predispose to pouch perforation. Perforations of gastro- or ileo-cystoplasties are rare, while colonic ones may be at greater risk [52, 53]. In a series from the USA, 21% of patients ruptured while drunk [54].

The diagnosis should always be suspected with sudden onset of abdominal pain and diminished drainage of urine on catheterisation. Examination usually shows the signs of peritonitis, but at first they may be minimal.

The best investigation is a CT scan (with a formal CT cystogram the most sensitive), but US may also show the pockets of free fluid that are characteristic of perforation (Figure 11.10) [55]. A fluoroscopic cystogram may appear normal even when the perforation is still open and can therefore give a false negative result [56]. Whatever form of cystogram is used, the patient should be positioned in a downward angle with adequate filling (assessed by using the maximum volume reported by the patient) and delayed images [56].

The treatment is to insert a catheter and establish free drainage. The lethal problem is septic shock which should always be anticipated. This requires immediate initiation of intravenous fluids, antibiotics and management in an intensive care unit. Unless there is improvement within a few hours, a laparotomy is essential to washout and drain the abdomen. It is not always necessary to close the perforation. If it is easily accessible,

Figure 11.10 Pre-contrast coronal and axial (a,b) images of the abdomen after perforation of a neobladder, showing extensive free fluid (ff). (c,d) Corresponding images after instillation of 150 mL dilute omnipaque into the neobladder (bl) in a CT cystogram: opacified urine is clearly seen outside the bladder and within the peritoneum. Note the more dilute contrast superiorly (arrow in d) as mixing is occurring. Contrast does not always leak out through the defect and so the cystogram can give a false negative result.

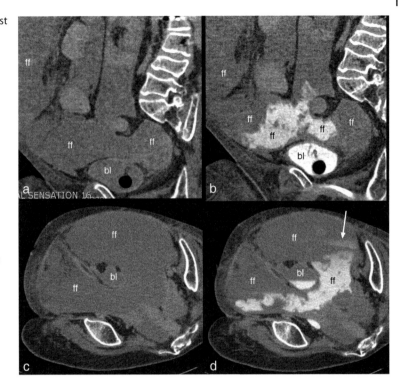

closure with a plug of omentum may be helpful, but free reservoir drainage, which should be continued for at least 3 weeks in all cases, will usually close it very well. There is often only a short window when the resuscitation has been achieved and before septic shock becomes irreversible, during which laparotomy is possible. The most common reason for a death with this diagnosis is delayed diagnosis and treatment so that this treatment window is missed.

Histological Changes

The spectrum of changes in the ileum is shown in Figure 11.11. Villous atrophy is seen at a mean of 4.9 years, a mixed pattern by 10.6 years and widespread subtotal change by 13 years. The range is very variable and different patterns of change may be seen after similar periods of exposure to urine. These changes are mirrored by the loss of folds seen on imaging (see Figures 6.10 and 9.10). This probably explains the relatively

small metabolic effects that are found with ileal reservoirs.

The bowel wall is infiltrated with inflammatory cells. The submucosa and muscularis are always thickened and splintered. The lymphatics are grossly dilated and the submucosa oedematous. Transitional epithelium grows in from the ureters over a radius of 3–5 mm, displacing the ileal epithelium and abnormal cells are found in the lining of conduits which have been labelled as dysplasia but there is no evidence that these are pre-neoplastic changes (Figure 11.12).

These changes have been widely reported in experimental animals and in human ileal conduits. The few reports of reservoir biopsies have shown a similar pattern, but the follow-up periods have been much shorter [57, 58]. It is most unlikely that these findings are an indication of malignant risk.

In colon used as a conduit, the mucosal pattern is not greatly changed from normal except that the goblet cells are decreased in size. There is a dense inflammatory infiltrate of plasma cells and eosinophils. These

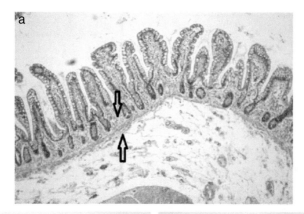

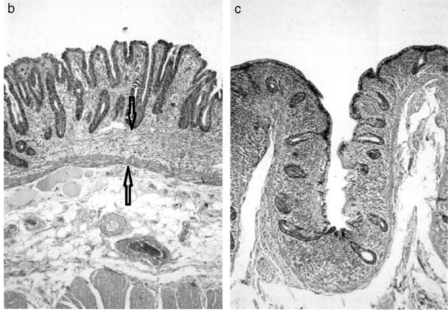

Figure 11.11 Photomicrographs with haematoxylin and eosin (H&E) staining showing: (a) normal ileal mucosa with long, spindly villi and thin submucosa (between the arrows); (b) partial villous atrophy the overall thickness of the mucosa is unchanged but the villi are shorter and the basal layer, containing the crypts of Lieberkuhn, is thicker (between the arrows); (c) subtotal atrophy is a more severe change in which the villi all but disappear and the mucosa takes on an appearance similar to colon.

changes are more marked with longer exposure to urine, and mitotic figures are seen with increasing frequency up to 15 years of follow-up. There is little information about the changes seen in colon reservoirs. Some inflammatory changes have been described, but in patients with a mean follow-up of only 9 years and 30% of patients had no changes at all [59].

In patients with a uretero-sigmoidostomy, sialomucin staining has been positive in biopsies close to the ureteric anastomosis in 90% of patients (Figure 11.13) [60]. In patients with ulcerative colitis, this would be considered a pre-malignant change. It may also be in the special situation of the uretero-sigmoidostomy which has a very high incidence of anastomotic malignancy. This change has not been reported in colocystoplasties. However, in rats with a colocystoplasty, non-invasive tumours occur in 20% after 2 years of follow-up [61].

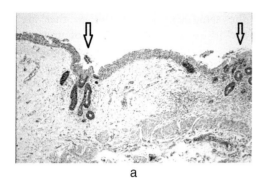

a

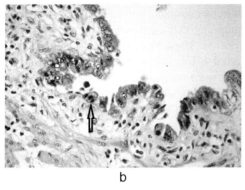

b

Figure 11.12 (a) In growth of transitional cell urothelium from the ureters (arrows). (b) Dysplastic cells (arrow), which are irregular, larger than usual and have bigger nuclei than the normal mucosal cells as in Figure 11.11(a).

Infection

In clinical practice, there is great difficulty in managing alleged urinary tract infections (UTI) in patients with intestinal reservoirs and conduits.

Reservoir infection is a diagnostic problem and symptoms can be non-specific. There may be malaise, low grade fever, feeling of a frequent need to empty the reservoir and other symptoms that are recognisable to individual patients. With a suspicious group of symptoms, a catheter specimen of urine should be sent for culture. The diagnosis depends on the culture of a single relevant organism. Blood tests are usually unhelpful, but the C-reacive protein (CRP) is occasionally raised. The critical issue is that, for a lower urinary tract infection to require antibiotics, it must be making the patient 'ill' in some way.

Acute pyelonephritis in a diverted patient is exactly the same as in anyone else. There is high fever, often with rigors, with pain and tenderness in the affected kidney. On investigation, the white blood count and CRP are raised. There is increasing use of more sophisticated biomarkers of infection such as procalcitonin or preseptin both for diagnosis and prognostication. US may show an oedematous kidney. Hydronephrosis will raise the possibility of a pyonephrosis.

With or without infection, a plain X-ray showing air in the upper tract, especially with a Mainz II, is an indication of reflux

Figure 11.13 Photomicrographs of biopsies from the colon stained with high iron diamine alcian blue. Left: from a normal colon showing dark staining of normal cells positive for sulfomucins. Right: from a uretero-sigmoidostomy showing blue staining in dysplastic cells positive for sialomucins.

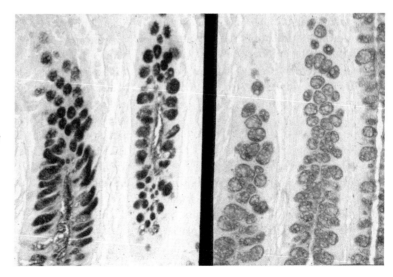

which will increase the risk of pyelonephritis (Figure 11.1).

It is particularly important to recognise that smelly urine on its own is not an indication for antibiotics. Gross, painless haematuria should not be ascribed to UTI, but is an indication to search for stones or cancer as it would in any other patient.

It is not surprising that UTI is greatly over-diagnosed. As with all other complications, the longer the follow-up, the higher the incidence becomes. With strict attention to diagnostic criteria, an incidence as low as 3% after a mean of 11 years has been reported [62]. Others give 8–11% at 5 years, which seems more probable.

With recurrent UTI, especially after a long period free of infection, it is prudent to look for reservoir stones. Although most will be identified on US, it may, occasionally, be necessary to perform a non-contrast CT scan. Review of catheterising technique may reveal that the reservoir is not being emptied completely or often enough.

Most urologists will try low dose prophylactic antibiotics such as nitrofurantoin or trimethoprim. With very persistent and poorly controlled recurrent UTI, twice weekly irrigation with gentamicin or chlorhexidine may be useful [63].

In a small series of 15 with the patients as their own pre-treatment controls, cranberry extract has been found to be a useful prophylactic. Before treatment all patients had persistent bacteriuria, though only 26% actually had symptomatic infection. Treatment was with 36 mg of the cranberry extract Urell®. There was only one positive culture over a mean of 18.5 months on treatment (6%) and no episodes of symptomatic UTI [64].

Neoplasia

Unlike those with a uretero-sigmoidostomy, patients whose urine is stored in isolated bowel segments or bladder augments have only a slightly increased risk of neoplasia in the long term.

The same nitroso compounds that are found in excess in the effluent of ureterosigmoidostomies are also found in urine from intestinal reservoirs. Levels are high when the urine contains bacteria and virtually disappear after antibiotic treatment [65]. Although it known that these compounds are carcinogens, there is no confirmation that they are responsible for cancers in intestinal reservoirs.

The majority of reservoir tumours are adenocarcinomas, but transitional cell and squamous cell carcinomas have also been reported. Higuchi *et al.* [66] recently concluded a long-term study of children who underwent augmentation cystoplasty and found no statistical difference in the malignancy rate in those augmented with ileum or colon versus control patients with the same diagnoses but no augmentation. However, their data suggest an increased risk of malignancy in patients with neurogenic bladder or exstrophy. Per decade, the risk of malignancy for ileal or colonic augmentation is 1.5%. It is uncertain whether this slightly increased incidence is a result of the intestinal reservoir or the underlying bladder abnormality. In a review of malignancies in German patients with augmentations, there was excess of chronic inflammatory conditions, particularly tuberculosis, in the bladder [67]. The risk of bladder cancer in patients with exstrophy is increased more than 600-fold at age 40 compared with the normal population [34].

There may be an increased risk of malignancy in gastro-cystoplasties. Where a denominator has been available, there have been five cases in 101 patients, 11–14 years postoperatively. All presented with metastases, four had died and one was alive with metastases at the time of publication [68]. The cumulative risk per decade at 2.8% is within the estimated rate for all forms of enteric bladder augmentation (1.5–5.5%) [69].

Unfortunately, most of the cases of malignancy in any reservoir that have been reported have developed in the interval between screening investigations. They are aggressive and rapidly fatal cancers. Neither surveillance endoscopy of the reservoir nor cytological examination of urine have been useful in their early detection [58]. Patients will usually present with symptoms and clinicians must investigate the standard indicators of bladder cancer such as haematuria urgently.

Urine Testing for Pregnancy

A chance observation has shown that the standard human chorionic gonadotrophin (HCG) antibody test for pregnancy (blue line test) is falsely positive on 57% of occasions in both women *and men* using urine from any intestinal reservoir. This may be only of passing interest in the latter; it is of critical importance in women. Those who wish to be pregnant may believe that they are suffering from recurrent miscarriage. Those who do not wish to be pregnant may be very distressed or even suicidal when finding a (false) positive. True pregnancy must be confirmed by measurement of the serum HCG [70].

The Conduit and Continence

The conduit is the weak link in the reconstruction chain. For a colorectal pouch, the anus is, by definition, the conduit and has already been considered. No complications directly related to passing urine through it have been reported. The native urethra is considered in Chapter 10. The other possible conduits are shown in the third column of Table 11.1.

Of these, there is general agreement that the appendix is the best. It is the easiest to harvest and to implant. It is resilient enough to survive catheterisation around six times a day for many years. Although there is a steadily rising complication rate as the years pass, particularly of stomal stenosis (25% in some series), surgical correction is usually possible. By 15 years of follow-up, about 8% will have to be re-made and 4% require correction of prolapse.

The Yang–Monti tube makes a good substitute when the appendix is not available. A series from France found that 94% were still in use at a mean of 5 years [71]. Conversely, in London it was found that 15 of 25 children (60%) had catheterisation difficulties. In seven of them it was caused by pouch-like aneurysms of the channel, a problem that is unique to the Monti. In this series, comparison was made with 69 contemporaneous appendix channels which had a 27% rate of difficulty with catheterisation. Other complications were similar between the two groups [72].

Data on the other types of catheterisable conduit are limited as numbers are small. Structures such as the ureter, detrusor, gastric or fallopian tubes have been used when more conventional options are not available. All are reported to be more complicated and less durable.

In a sense, a part of all catheterisable channels is a skin tube – the point where the channel reaches the surface. It may be a fashioned tube or the umbilicus. The highest complication rate comes from stenosis at this anastomosis. The longer the follow-up, the greater is the rate. It can never be said that enough time has passed that risk is eliminated.

The VQZ anastomosis devised by Ransley is said to have the lowest stenosis rate, but there have been no formal comparisons. In a retrospective series, there were no stenoses with a VQZ, while 45% of skin tubes and 25% of umbilical stomas developed stenosis. These data are not very robust as there were only eight patients with VQZ and their follow-up was only up to 3 years. The patients with a skin tube had been followed for up to 6 years and the umbilical ones to 14 years [73]. It is unlikely to be immune from stenosis in the long term.

It is almost always possible to make a reservoir with a catheterisable stoma continent with current standard techniques. With buried tubes using the Mitrofanoff principle, continence is reported in 90–100% of patients even beyond 15 years of follow-up. In 100 consecutive patients with widely varying types of continent suprapubic reconstructions, we found no statistically significant difference in the continence rate with any combination of reservoir or conduit [74, 75].

In patients who have been reliably continent but after a long interval become incontinent, three possibilities should be considered.

1 The continence mechanism, especially of a buried tube such as the Mitrofanoff, has deteriorated. The buried tube can be reconstructed fairly easily at operation. A failed natural urethral sphincter is almost impossible to correct unless an artificial urinary sphincter can be used. It is usually necessary to close off the bladder neck, above the prostate in males, and implant a suprapubic continence channel.

2 The pouch has become unstable. This is rare and will be diagnosed on urodynamic testing. Further augmentation will usually correct the problem.

3 Progressive damage and scarring has caused a structural change in the reservoir. This is also uncommon, and may be the result of a poorly constructed reservoir. It is a particular problem when the bladder is augmented and the anastomosis is an inadequate 'clam'. It is then quite easy for progressive scarring to form an hourglass deformity and the lower, bladder, compartment reverts to instability and hence incontinence (see Figure 9.10). Proper re-formation of the clam resolves the problem.

References

1 Nabi G, Yong SM, Ong E, McPherson G, Grant A, N'Dow J. Is orthotopic bladder replacement the new gold standard? Evidence from a systematic review. *J Urol.* 2005; 174: 21–28.

2 Blackburn SC, Parkar S, Prime M, *et al.* Ileal bladder augmentation and vitamin B12: levels decrease with time after surgery. *J Pediatr Urol.* 2012; 8(1): 47–50.

3 Rosenbaum DH, Cain MP, Kaefer M, *et al.* Ileal enterocystoplasty and B12 deficiency in pediatric patients. *J Urol.* 2008; 179(4): 1544–1547.

4 Einarsson K. Metabolic effects caused by exclusion of intestinal segments. *Scand J Urol Nephrol.* 1992; 142(Suppl.): 21–26.

5 Canning DA, Perman JA, Jeffs RD, Gearhart JP. Nutritional consequences of bowel segments in the lower urinary tract. *J Urol.* 1989; 142: 509–511.

6 N'Dow J, Leung HY, Marshall C, Neal DE. Bowel dysfunction after bladder reconstruction. *J Urol.* 1998; 159: 1470–1475.

7 Somani BK, Kumar V, Wong S, *et al.* Bowel dysfunction after transposition of intestinal segments into the urinary tract: 8-year prospective cohort study. *J Urol.* 2007; 177(5): 1793–1798.

8 Shridhar KN, Samuells CT, Woodhouse CRJ. Glucose absorption from urinary conduits. *Br Med J.* 1983; 287: 1327–1329.

9 Hayward RH, Wakim KG, Remine WH, Grindlay JH. An experimental study of the role of the colonic mucosa in hyperchloraemic acidosis. *Surg Gynecol Obstet.* 1961; 112: 357–365.

10 Ghoneim MA. The recto-sigmoid bladder for urinary diversion. *Br J Urol.* 1970; 42: 429–433.

11 Nurse DE, Mundy AR. Metabolic complications of cystoplasty. *Br J Urol.* 1989; 63: 165–170.

12 McConnell JB, Murison J, Stewart WK. The role of the colon in the pathogenesis of hyperchloraemic acidosis in ureterosigmoid anastomosis. *Clin Sci.* 1979; 57: 305–312.

13 Boddy K, King PC, Stewart WK, Flemming LW. Whole body potassium in patients with ureterosigmoid anastomoses. *Br J Urol.* 1975; 47: 277–282.

14 Madsen PO. The etiology of hyperchloraemic acidosis following intestinal anastomosis: an experimental study. *J Urol.* 1964; 92: 448–454.

15 Gerharz EW, Mosekilde L, Thomsen JS, Gasser JA, Moniz C, Woodhouse CRJ. The effect of enterocystoplasty on bone strength assessed at four different skeletal sites in a rat model. *Bone.* 2003; 33: 549–556.

16 McDougal WS, Koch MO, Shands C, Price RR. Boney demineralisation following urinary intestinal diversion. *J Urol.* 1988; 140: 853–855.

17 Gerharz EW, Gasser J, Moniz C, Ransley PG, Reidmiller H, Woodhouse CRJ. Skeletal growth and long term bone over after enterocystoplasty in the rat model. *Br J Urol.* 1998; 81(Suppl. 4): 28.

18 Abes M, Sarihan H, Madenci E. Evaluation of bone mineral density with dual x-ray absorptiometry for osteoporosis in children with bladder augmentation. *J Pediatr Surg.* 2003; 38(2): 230–232.

19 Jacobs A, Barr-Stirling W. The late results of ureterocolic anastomosis. *Br J Urol.* 1952; 24: 259–316.

20 Harrison AR. Clinical and metabolic observations on osteomalacia following ureterosigmoidostomy. *Br J Urol.* 1958; 30: 453–462.

21 Ronholt C, Rasmussen OO, Christiansen J. Ambulatory manometric recording of anorectal activity. *Dis Colon Rectum.* 1999; 42(12): 1551–1559.

22 Dall FH, Jorgensen CS, Houe D, Gregersen H, Djurhuus JC. Biomechanical wall properties of the human rectum: a study with impedance planimetry. *Gut.* 1993; 34(11): 1581–1586.

23 Jones MA, Breckman B, Hendry WF. Life with an ileal conduit: results of questionaire surveys of patients and urological surgeons. *Br J Urol.* 1980; 52: 21–25.

24 Gumus E, Miroglu C, Saporta L, *et al.* Rectodynamic and radiological assessment in modified Mainz pouch II cases. *Eur Urol.* 2000; 38(3): 316–322.

25 Woodhouse CRJ. The place of the augmented rectal pouch in urinary diversion. *BJU Int.* 2004; 94: 756–758.

26 Szucs M, Keszthelyi A, Szendroi A, *et al.* Investigation of anal sphincter function following Mainz pouch type II urinary diversion after radical cystectomy. *Int Urol Nephrol.* 2012; 44(4): 1013–1020.

27 Hammer E. Cancer du colon sigmoide dix ans apres implantation des ureteres d'une vessie exstrphiee. *J Urol (Paris).* 1929; 28: 260–263.

28 Stewart M. Urinary diversion and bowel cancer. *Ann R Coll Surg.* 1986; 68: 98–102.

29 Strachan JR, Matthews JNS, Rees HC, Cooke T. Kinetic changes in experimental colonic urinary diversion. *Br J Surg.* 1987; 74: 1046–1048.

30 Pitluk H, Poticha SM. Carcinoma of the colon and rectum in patients less than 40 years of age. *Surg Gynecol Obstet.* 1983; 157(4): 335–337.

31 Austen M, Kalble T. Secondary malignancies in different forms of urinary diversion using isolated gut. *J Urol.* 2004; 172: 831–838.

32 Strachan JR, Woodhouse CRJ. Malignancy following ureterosigmoidostomy in patients with exstrophy. *Br J Surg.* 1991; 78: 1216–1218.

33 Greenwell TJ, Woodhams SD, Smalley T, Mundy AR. Effect of antibiotics on enterocystoplasty urinary nitrosamine levels. *Urology.* 2001; 58(5): 660–664.

34 Smeulders N, Woodhouse CRJ. Neoplasia in adult exstrophy patients. *BJU Int.* 2001; 87: 623–628.

35 Cairns SR, Scholefield JH, Steele RJ, *et al.* Guidelines for colorectal cancer screening and surveillance in moderate and high risk groups (update from 2002). *Gut.* 2010; 59: 666–690.

36 Spence HM, Hoffman WW, Fosmire GP. Tumour of the colon as a late complication of ureterosigmoidostomy for exstrophy of the bladder. *Br J Urol.* 1979; 51:466–470.

37 Woodhouse CRJ. Lower urinary tract replacement and reconstruction. *Adolescent Urology and Long-term Outcomes.* Oxford: Wiley Blackwell, 2015: 91–116.

38 Chen Z, Lu G, Li X, *et al.* Better compliance contributes to better nocturnal continence with orthotopic ileal neobladder than ileocolonic neobladder after radical cystectomy for bladder cancer. *Urology.* 2009; 73(4): 838–843.

39 Schrier BP, Laguna MP, van der PF, Isorna S, Witjes JA. Comparison of orthotopic sigmoid and ileal neobladders: continence and urodynamic parameters. *Eur Urol.* 2005; 47(5): 679–685.

40 Kronner KM, Casale AJ, Cain MP, Zerin MJ, Keating MA, Rink RC. Bladder calculi in the pediatric augmented bladder. *J Urol.* 1998; 160: 1096–1098.

41 Hamid R, Robertson WG, Woodhouse CRJ. Comparison of biochemistry and diet in patients with enterocystoplasty who do and do not form stones. *BJU Int.* 2008; 101: 1427–1432.

42 Nurse DE, McInerney PD, Thomas PJ, Mundy AR. Stones in enterocystoplasties. *Br J Urol.* 1996; 77: 684–687.

43 Terai A, Ueda T, Kakehi Y, *et al.* Urinary calculi as a late complication of the Indiana continent urinary diversion: comparison with the Kock pouch procedure. *J Urol.* 1996; 155: 66–68.

44 Robertson WG. A risk factor model of stone-formation. *Front Biosci.* 2003; 8: s1330–s1338.

45 Khoury AE, Salomon M, Doche R, *et al.* Stone formation after augmentation cystoplasty: the role of intestinal mucus. *J Urol.* 1997; 158: 1133–1137.

46 Barrosso U, Jednak R, Fleming P, Barthold JS, Gonzalez R. Bladder calculi in children who perform clean intermittent catheterisation. *BJU Int.* 2000; 85: 879–884.

47 Woodhouse CRJ, Lennon GM. Management and aetiology of stones in intestinal urinary reservoirs. *Br J Urol.* 1998; 81(Suppl. 4): 47.

48 Woodhouse CRJ, Lennon GM. Management and aetiology of stones in intestinal urinary reservoirs in adolescents. *Eur Urol.* 2001; 39: 253–259.

49 Harraz AM, Mosbah A, El Assmy A, Gad H, Shaaban AA. Renal function evaluation in patients undergoing orthotopic bladder substitution: a systematic review of literature. *BJU Int.* 2014; 114(4): 484–495.

50 Mansson W, Bakke A, Bergman B, *et al.* Perforation of continent urinary reservoirs: Scandinavian experience. *Scand J Urol Nephrol.* 1997; 31(6): 529–532.

51 Bauer SB, Hendren WH, Kozakewich H, *et al.* Perforation of the augmented bladder. *J Urol.* 1992; 148: 699–703.

52 Rink RC, Hollensbe DW, Adams MC, Keating MA. Is sigmoid enterocystoplasty at greatest risk for perforation? Observations and etiology in 23 bladder perforations in 264 patients. *Scand J Urol Nephrol.* 1992; 142(Suppl.): 179.

53 DeFoor W, Tackett L, Minevich E, Wacksman J, Sheldon C. Risk factors for spontaneous bladder perforation after augmentation cystoplasty. *Urology.* 2003; 62(4): 737–741.

54 Fox JA, Husmann DA. Continent urinary diversion in childhood: complications of alcohol abuse developing in adulthood. *J Urol.* 2010; 183: 2342–2346.

55 Han KS, Choi HJ, Jung DC, *et al.* A prospective evaluation of conventional cystography for detection of urine leakage at the vesicourethral anastomosis site after radical prostatectomy based on computed tomography. *Clin Radiol.* 2011; 66(3): 251–256.

56 Singh S, Choong S. Rupture and perforation of urinary reservoirs made from bowel. *World J Urol.* 2004; 22(3): 222–226.

57 Gitlin JS, Wu XR, Sun TT, Ritchey ML, Shapiro E. New concepts of histological changes in experimental augmentation

cystoplasty: insights into the development of neoplastic transformation at the enterovesical and gastrovesical anastomosis. *J Urol*. 1999; 162(3 Pt 2): 1096–1100.

58 Hamid R, Greenwell TJ, Nethercliffe J, Freeman A, Venn S, Woodhouse CRJ. Routine surveillance cystoscopy for patients with augmentation and substitution cystoplasty for benign urological conditions: is it necessary? *BJU Int.*2009; 104: 392–397.

59 Vajda P, Kaiser L, Magyarlaki T, Farkas A, Vastyan AM, Pinter AB. Histological findings after colocystoplasty and gastrocystoplasty. *J Urol*. 2002; 168(2): 698–701.

60 Silverman SH, Woodhouse CR, Strachan JR, Cumming J, Keighley MR. Long-term management of patients who have had urinary diversions into colon. *Br J Urol*. 1986; 58(6): 634–639.

61 Little JS Jr, Klee LW, Hoover DM, Rink RC. Long-term histopathological changes observed in rats subjected to augmentation cystoplasty. *J Urol*. 1994; 152(2 Pt 2): 720–724.

62 Lopez PP, Moreno Valle JA, Espinosa L, *et al*. Enterocystoplasty in children with neuropathic bladders: long-term follow-up. *J Pediatr Urol*. 2008; 4(1): 27–31.

63 Traxel E, DeFoor W, Minevich E, *et al*. Low incidence of urinary tract infections following renal transplantation in children with bladder augmentation. *J Urol*. 2011; 186(2): 667–671.

64 Botto H, Neuzillet Y. Effectiveness of a cranberry (*Vaccinium macrocarpon*) preparation in reducing asymptomatic bacteriuria in patients with an ileal enterocystoplasty. *Scand J Urol Nephrol*. 2010; 44(3): 165–168.

65 Woodhams SD, Greenwell TJ, Smalley T, Mundy AR. Factors causing variation in urinary N-nitrosamine levels in enterocystoplasties. *BJU Int*. 2001; 88(3): 187–191.

66 Higuchi TT, Granberg CF, Fox JA, Husmann DA. Augmentation cystoplasty and risk of neoplasia: fact, fiction and controversy. *J Urol*. 2010; 184: 2492–2497.

67 Kalble T, Hofmann I, Riedmiller H, Vergho D. Tumor growth in urinary diversion: a multicenter analysis. *Eur Urol*. 2011; 60(5): 1081–1086.

68 Castellan M, Gosalbez R, Bar-Yosef Y, Labbie A. Complications after use of gastric segments for lower urinary tract reconstruction. *J Urol*. 2012; 187(5): 1823–1827.

69 Vermulakonda VM, Lendvay TS, Shnorhavorian M, *et al*. Metastatic adenocarcinoma after augmentation gastrocystoplasty. *J Urol*. 2008; 179: 1094–1097.

70 Nakhal RS, Wood D, Woodhouse C, Creighton SM. False-positive pregnancy tests following enterocystoplasty. *Br J Obstet Gynaecol*. 2011; 119(3): 366–368.

71 Lemelle JL, Simo AK, Schmitt M. Comparative study of the Yang–Monti channel and appendix for continent diversion in the Mitrofanoff and Malone principles. *J Urol*. 2004; 172(5 Pt 1): 1907–1910.

72 Narayanaswamy B, Wilcox DT, Cuckow PM, Duffy PG, Ransley PG. The Yang–Monti ileovesicostomy: a problematic channel? *BJU Int*. 2001; 87(9): 861–865.

73 Landau EH, Gofrit ON, Cipele H, *et al*. Superiority of the VQZ over the tubularized skin flap and the umbilicus for continent abdominal stoma in children. *J Urol*. 2008; 180(4 Suppl): 1761–1765.

74 Woodhouse CRJ, MacNeilly AE. The Mitrofanoff principle: expanding on a versatile theme. *Br J Urol*. 1994; 74: 447–453.

75 Harris CF, Cooper CS, Hutcheson JC, Snyder HM 3rd., Appendicovesicostomy: the mitrofanoff procedure-a 15-year perspective. *J Urol*. 2000; 163(6): 1922–1926.

12

Surgery on the Benign Prostate

Doug Pendse and Mark R. Feneley

Introduction

Research since the 1970s has shown that the lower urinary tract symptoms (LUTS), once described as 'prostatism', have several causes, one of which is bladder outflow obstruction (BOO) resulting from benign prostatic enlargement (BPE). Diagnostic imaging is used selectively in the assessment of men with LUTS, alongside clinical assessment of symptoms and urinary flow tests [1]. Although the most common cause of LUTS in men is BPE, the diagnosis is often multifactorial and the first role of imaging is to evaluate for other potential causes of voiding dysfunction. A second role of imaging is to identify complications of BPE such as bladder calculi, hydronephrosis and urinary retention. Baseline imaging tests in men with LUTS have useful prognostic value, for those considering either medical [2–8] or surgical [9, 10] treatment options and are important for selecting and counselling patients for surgery. Lastly, in those patients in whom surgery is undertaken, imaging can be useful for both pre-operative planning and follow-up (Table 12.1).

In uncomplicated cases, without urinary retention, no further structural assessment is typically carried out until endoscopic examination at the time of surgical intervention. Assuming that BPE is determined to be the cause of symptoms, medical and surgical treatments are available. If the former is selected, it is particularly important that imaging studies are completed as endoscopy is not a part of the management.

Although knowledge of prostatic size is important, more detailed structural imaging of the prostate is rarely undertaken for the purpose of refining surgical treatment. While different operative techniques may be favoured according to size, that itself does not indicate the need for treatment; however, it does contribute to risk of clinical progression and future need for surgical treatment [11].

When there is a history of pelvic injury or peripheral neurological disease, patients should be fully investigated before surgery as BOO is only one of several possible causes.

Procedures

There is a large and growing number of treatment modalities for BPE, wherein the position of transurethral resection of the prostate (TURP) as the 'gold standard' continues to be debated [12–15]. Just as structural conformation of the prostate and bladder neck may be relevant to assessment of symptoms, it may also be relevant to the applicability of some treatment modalities. Most operative treatments aim to debulk the prostate, by removing the median and lateral lobes, as evident endoscopically,

Radiology and Follow-up of Urologic Surgery, First Edition. Edited by Christopher Woodhouse and Alex Kirkham.
© 2018 John Wiley & Sons Ltd. Published 2018 by John Wiley & Sons Ltd.

Table 12.1 Role of investigations in the diagnostic evaluation of bladder outflow obstruction (BOO) and benign prostatic enlargement (BPE).

Test	Suggested role	Comments
Urinary flow rate	Routine in all patients	
PVR	Routine in all patients	US preferred to catheterisation
Symptomatic assessment tools (i.e. AUA-7, IPSS)	Routine in all patients	
Bladder US	In selected patients depending on availability	Can be combined with PVR and uro-flow tests (USCD)
TRUS	In selected patients as part of pre-operative planning	Pvol assessment (abdominal or TRUS) may be useful in planning medical therapy
Upper tract imaging (renal US)	For investigation of complications of BPE	Haematuria, renal dysfunction, calculi, high PVR or UTI
Urodynamics/VCMG	In patients refractory to treatment	May be useful in pre-operative planning in selected cases (i.e. to exclude underactive bladder)
Urethrogram	In patients with suspected urethral stricture	Ascending and descending (voiding) studies
Multiparametric prostate MRI	Not recommended for assessment of BPE	Reserve for assessment of prostate carcinoma

AUA, American Urological Association; IPSS, International Prostate Symptom Score; MRI, magnetic resonance imaging; Pvol, prostate volume; PVR, post-void residual; TRUS, transrectal ultrasound of prostate; US, ultrasound; USCD, ultrasound cysto-dynamogram; UTI, urinary tract infection; VCMG, video-cystometrogram.

with techniques of resection, vaporisation (whether electrical or laser), or enucleation or combinations as vaporesection or vapor enuculeation. For the smaller prostate, transurethral incision of the prostate or bladder neck remain worthwhile and less invasive alternatives [16–18]. Whilst sharing the same therapeutic principle, there are numerous combinations of technique and modality, but currently many of them are not approved outside research evaluation owing to limited high quality evidence and long-term outcome data.

Debulking may be important where relief of obstruction relies on removal of tissue. The amount of tissue clearance may be subject to the limitations of the surgical modality in larger prostates. Regardless of procedure-specific limitations, tissue clearance needs to be sufficient for relief of obstruction as this likely relates to all-important surgical outcomes including magnitude and durability of benefit. Unfortunately, no volumetric data exist that describe this relationship for any given modality; however, inference can be gained from comparative studies. Evaluation of TURP against holmium enucleation (HoLep) in a randomised study indicates that HoLep removes more tissue with better relief of obstruction and subsequently has a lower re-operation rate [19]. By contrast, many minimally invasive treatments have been compared with TURP, demonstrating less effective tissue removal and higher re-operation rates. Nevertheless, at least in smaller prostates, minimally invasive treatments are often sufficiently effective, particularly where tissue clearance may not necessarily be required for excellent outcomes.

Aside from consideration of relative effects on sexual function and complications, voiding outcomes after minimally invasive treatments may be overall less durable as evidenced by higher re-operation rates, emphasising the urodynamic importance of relieving obstruction. In a recent prospective non-randomised volumetric study, laser vaporisation was shown to be less effective than TURP for tissue removal, for improvement in uroflow and prostate-specific antigen (PSA) reduction, and was associated with a higher re-operation rate, significant in larger prostates measuring more than 40 mL [20]. Whilst it is beyond the remit of this chapter to review the multitude of therapeutic interventions, it is surprising that a standard measurement of volume is not more frequently taken into account in considering the alternative treatment options.

Approaches to destroy prostate tissue in situ have had variable success. They appeal as minimally invasive and therefore office-based procedures, or on account of side-effect profile, sometimes outweighing regulatory recommendations and lack of data on longer term outcomes. Examples include interstitial laser, transurethral needle ablation (TUNA), transurethral microwave therapy (TUMT), transurethral ethanol ablation of the prostate (TEAP) and, more recently, Rezūm therapy. Those having little impact on prostate volume probably depend in part on changes in neuromuscular function within the prostate and bladder neck for – often limited – therapeutic efficacy. Procedures that mechanically open the prostatic urethra without changing prostate volume have included prostatic balloon dilatation, abandoned for high failure and complication rates, and prostatic stents, now infrequently considered other than in a surgical high-risk or palliative setting on account of disappointing durability.

A relatively new treatment, now approved with good evidence for durable benefit, is the urethral lift procedure (UroLift™). It achieves efficacy by displacing the lateral lobes to relieve endo-prostatic obstruction without compromising bladder neck function or causing prostate tissue damage; thereby sexual function is also preserved (Figure 12.1). Another minimally invasive

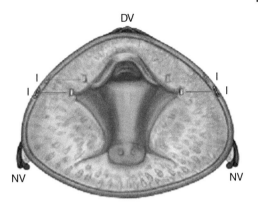

Figure 12.1 Schematic diagram showing Urolift™ implants (I) after their deployment, in relation to the dorsal vein (DV) and neurovascular bundles (NV). Image courtesy of Justin Hall, Vice President and General Manager EMEA NeoTract®, Inc.

option attracting interest for treating large prostates is selective arterial embolisation, particularly where invasive surgical options are contraindicated; however, embolisation is not approved outside research evaluation.

Published literature that focuses on outcomes of surgery for large prostates aims to demonstrate feasibility or otherwise of specific technologies and techniques, along with procedure-specific risks and complications. Successful outcome also emphasises surgical skill and experience; it would be simplistic to surmise that necessary skills for any multitude of procedures are ubiquitous among surgeons. Whilst there are many technical surgical factors other than prostate size that determine outcome and complications, size might be an objective leveller in the appropriateness of technologies as well as for evaluation of outcomes [21].

Outcomes and Complications

When a patient is satisfied with the outcome of his operation, follow-up investigations are not needed. However, a measure of urine flow rate and post-void residual provide objective confirmation of the patient's opinion. In practice, men who are satisfied with the outcome of surgery are discharged.

Surgical procedures are nonetheless subject to complications and outcomes that reflect the effects of surgery on voiding and sexual function relative to pre-existing status and the indications for surgery. Significant perioperative complications include capsular perforation, bleeding and need for blood transfusion, electrolyte disturbance leading to metabolic syndrome, infection and sepsis [22]. Procedure-specific perioperative risks relate to the surgical modality, operative procedure and duration, and composition of irrigation fluid, and usually they are less for minimally invasive procedures than TURP.

Postoperative Failure to Void

Following an otherwise successful prostate procedure, normal voiding may not occur on initial catheter removal in around 10% of cases. The first consideration is usually whether an adequate operation has been carried out. The removal of a previously protrusive median lobe and formation of a central prostate cavity may be evident on ultrasound (US). However, the apparent size of the prostate defect may be affected by the degree of bladder filling and mechanical characteristics of the prostate; similarly, the relative size of the prostate after surgery needs to take into consideration the cavity size and the weight of tissue removed. The effect of successful surgery on median lobe protrusion is shown in Figure 12.2, and on prostate volume for a different patient in Figure 12.3. In practice, whatever the conclusion of a postoperative US, failure to void usually requires re-catheterisation and further trials without catheter (TWOC). Re-establishment of voiding without the need for a further procedure may take up to 3 months.

Continued Failure to Void or Unsatisfactory Voiding

Invasive investigations, including video-urodynamic and cystoscopic evaluation, are needed when treatment outcomes remain unsatisfactory, particularly when the most

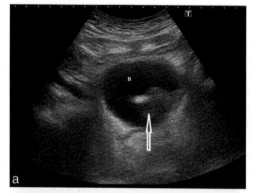

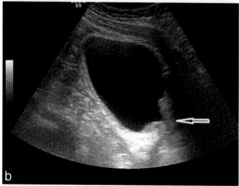

Figure 12.2 (a) Sagittal transabdominal ultrasound (US) of the bladder demonstrating a large median lobe of prostate (arrow) in patient with benign prostatic enlargement (BPE). B, bladder. (b) Sagittal transabdominal US of the bladder in the same patient following thulium vaporesection of the prostate. The median lobe is no longer present and the bladder neck is open at rest (arrow).

obvious cause – chronic retention – is shown on US (Figure 12.4). Even in less extreme cases of post-surgical voiding dysfunction, non-invasive assessments such as urine flow rate and post-void residual do not usually have the value for assessment of the cause as they would in the untreated setting. However, these investigations may be included for comparison with pre-treatment tests, and are necessary to secure a robust salvage therapeutic strategy.

In some cases, factors contributing to unsatisfactory surgical outcomes such as overactive bladder (OAB) may have existed pre-operatively; OAB may contribute to postoperative urinary incontinence alongside

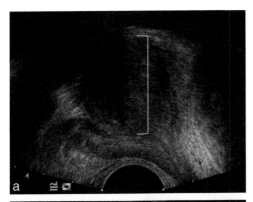

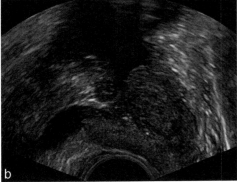

Figure 12.3 (a) Sagittal transrectal ultrasound scan (TRUS) of the prostate demonstrating hypertrophy of the transitional zone (callipers) in a patient with BPE. Overall prostate volume is 60 mL. (b) Sagittal TRUS in same patient following treatment with thulium vaporesection. There is significant volume reduction of transition zone seen on TRUS with an open bladder neck. Overall prostate volume is now 30 mL.

reduced outflow resistance. OAB secondary to obstruction causing frequency and urgency may take several months to settle, and otherwise may require secondary medical or surgical treatment.

Inadequate emptying may be the result of pre-existing bladder diverticula (Figure 12.5). Most surgeons will deal with proven bladder outflow obstruction first and reconsider the role of the diverticula afterwards. Diverticula have no muscle in the wall and may act as a 'blow-off', preventing the generation of sufficient detrusor pressure to achieve emptying. They may also act as sumps from which the true bladder re-fills, giving an early sensation of the need for a repeat void.

This, and other complications such as stones or recurrent infection, will require removal of the diverticula and reconstitution of the detrusor after the prostatectomy.

Surgery sometimes fails in its purpose, even when a procedure is performed as intended and technically correctly [23]. In standard clinical practice, chronic retention may persist reflecting an underactive bladder rather than failure to relieve obstruction; in such circumstances, prostate surgery may well still have been indicated, albeit with an inherent but often unevaluated increased risk of failure [24]. In the absence of a definitive indication such as retention, surgery for low pressure non-obstructed voiding may often not restore adequate voiding, and should be considered carefully.

In some situations, the primary procedure may have been insufficient to adequately relieve outflow obstruction. That conclusion is intuitive where there is persistent urinary retention until a second procedure proves successful in restoring voiding. Retrospectively, the adequacy of the surgery or the choice of procedure may be challenged: was the initial operation adequate or was the procedure unsuitable for the debulking required? These considerations are often debated when comparing outcomes among different modalities; however, evidence for adequate volume reduction for any given procedure, based on studies of long-term outcomes, remains scant [25].

Cystoscopy is invariable necessary where surgical outcomes are unsatisfactory to reassess the prostate, and to detect urethral stricture or bladder neck stenosis requiring re-operation. Residual prostatic tissue or new growth may cause obstruction of the prostatic urethra or form a prolapsing ball valve at the bladder neck. The presence of residual obstructing tissue in this situation has entirely different implications for relieving LUTS than where there is no obstruction and further surgery will not be beneficial.

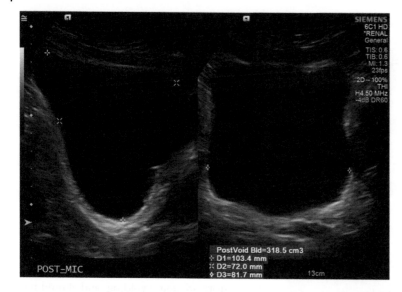

Figure 12.4 Transabdominal bladder US, sagittal image on left, axial image on right. The study shows a post-voiding residual volume of 318.5 mL.

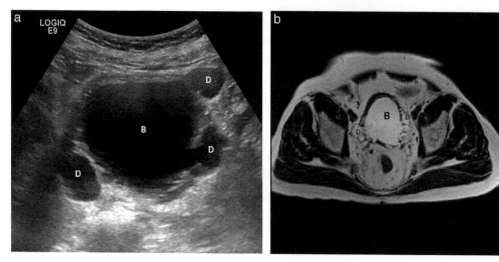

Figure 12.5 (a) Axial transabdominal US of the bladder (B) showing marked bladder wall trabeculation with diverticula (D). (b) Axial pelvic magnetic resonance imaging (MRI) of same patient (T2-weighted image).

Sexual Function

Ejaculatory dysfunction attributed to retrograde ejaculation or anejaculation is a common sequela of prostate surgery and the main cause of subsequent sexual dissatisfaction. It occurs in around 75% of patients after TURP [26]. Patients should be warned of its likelihood but it cannot be regarded as a true complication. It may be less common with treatments that are minimally invasive, parallel to which they also might be considered less effective [27, 28]. The cause might be understood when a prostate cavity is seen underneath an open bladder neck; however, other anatomical factors may enable ejaculation to be preserved in spite of bladder neck disruption (Figure 12.2b) [27–30]. In contrast, the apparently similar effect of alpha-blockade may include central inhibition of ejaculation alongside any effect on the bladder neck allowing true retrograde emission.

Surgical treatments that aim to maintain ejaculatory function do so by surgically preserving the so-called ejaculatory zone of the prostate adjacent to the veru montanum and paracollicular region irrespective of bladder neck function [31]. Procedures such as the urethral lift maintain sexual function, and avoid tissue destruction or manipulation of the bladder neck (Figure 12.6). Indications for urethral lift include absence of a protruding median lobe (as this cannot be displaced from its obstructive position) and a prostate that is not excessively enlarged.

Erectile dysfunction after prostatectomy for BPE has been a contentious subject for many years. About 12% of all patients are said to experience deterioration in erectile function according to recent literature; however, a similar percentage report improvement after surgery [32]. There are few prospective studies on men aimed specifically at determining the incidence related to surgery, and those that exist have conflicting results. In untreated patients erectile function deteriorates with age irrespective of co-morbidities [22, 33]. Favilla *et al.* [34] reported that the International Index of Erectile Function-5 score (IIEF-5) in 178 sexually active patients fell from a mean of 24 (normal erectile function) to 18 (mild erectile dysfunction) at 1 year after TURP which had a *p* value of <0.0001. However, this mean

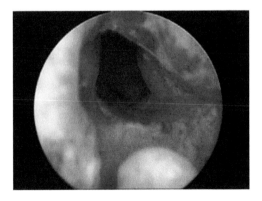

Figure 12.6 Prostatic urethra after Urethral Lift Procedure. Image courtesy of Justin Hall, Vice President and General Manager EMEA NeoTract®, Inc.

disguised the facts that 60% maintained their pre-operative IIEF-5 score and 40% even maintained antegrade ejaculation.

A more interesting prospective study has been reported by Mishriki *et al.* [35] of a 12-year follow-up of the sexual function in men after TURP corroborated by their sexual partners. All of the 73 men who were sexually active before surgery remained the same at 6 months of follow-up (47 men were not followed up). Of the men who were impotent pre-operatively, 15% resumed sexual activity postoperatively. At 6 years, 31 of 101 patients (31%) who completed the sexual function questionnaire were still active and the same percentage was found at 12 years.

Postoperative erectile dysfunction in men with prior normal erectile function is more likely in men with diabetes, hypertension, higher cardiac risk index, age over 65 and a high transfusion rate perioperatively [36]. The extent of surgery does not seem to impact on its incidence, whereas capsular perforation may do so [32]. The type of energy used to debulk the prostate does not appear to make any difference to the risk. Conventional mono-polar and bi-polar TURP have been compared prospectively in a randomised trial with no difference in outcome [37]. Literature review suggests no consistent difference with laser surgeries, minimally invasive treatments including TUMT, TUNA and ethanol ablation compared to TURP [28, 38]. Even a traditional open prostatectomy has no different outcome from TURP [36]. The risk associated with minimally invasive treatments may be less for a variety of reasons that also reflect non-surgical factors. Among these, GreenLight™ laser appears not to reduce sexual function except in those who already have an IIEF-5 score of less than 19 [39, 40].

This subject needs detailed discussion with the patient and, if possible, his partner to avoid disappointment for the patient and potential litigation for the surgeon.

Incontinence

Urinary incontinence after prostate surgery reflects bladder and sphincter dysfunction and their coordination, assuming normal underlying neurology. Many cases resolve after physiological adaptation of the bladder to lower outflow resistance, and spontaneous resolution of postoperative irritative symptoms by healing, sometimes facilitated by pelvic floor exercises and antimuscarinic medication. Underlying this, bladder outflow obstruction may be reversibly contributory to bladder instability prior to surgery, though there may be other non-reversible factors affecting bladder function including functional capacity and compliance, with age and duration of symptoms also playing a part. Other causes of incontinence include sphincter weakness from surgical injury which is relatively rare, mixed urge and stress incontinence, or residual obstruction from adenoma, bladder neck stenosis or stricture. For an adequate functional assessment, video-urodynamic studies and cystoscopy are essential in discriminating between these factors. The same considerations apply prior to surgery when there is a history of pelvic injury or peripheral neurological disease, which should have been investigated pre-operatively.

Stricture

Bladder neck stenosis or urethral stricture may develop at any time after lower urinary tract surgery. Vascular factors or previous injury may predispose, and frequently would not be evident pre-operatively. Duration of the surgical procedure and endoscopic sheath size may be contributory to comparative differences in stricture rate among modalities. These complications may be heralded by recurrent symptoms of obstruction, to be distinguished from the effect of residual obstructing prostatic tissue or subsequent regrowth. They would usually be diagnosed by urethro-cystoscopy, otherwise by urethrographic imaging (Figure 12.7) or video-cystometrography (VCMG) (see Chapter 14).

VCMG is particularly valuable for guiding management of LUTS persisting after surgery. However, even in this situation, it cannot provide an absolute prediction of surgical outcome. While there may be a place for cystometry prior to the initial surgery, not least for guiding the recommendation of surgery itself [41], other symptomatic and clinical considerations guided by standard non-invasive functional investigations, including uroflow and post-void residual, may be a sufficiently pragmatic strategy [42, 43].

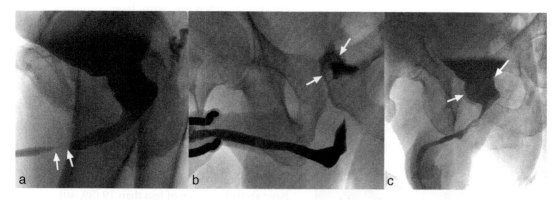

Figure 12.7 (a) A descending urethrogram showing a bulbar stricture (arrows) 1 year after transurethral resection of the prostate (TURP). This was treated by a formal urethroplasty, and on (b) ascending and (c) descending studies 3 months later the bulbar stricture is no longer seen. Small nodules of residual or recurrent BPE are seen best on the ascending study (b, arrows), before the prostatic fossa is fully distended. On the descending study (c) the open bladder neck is easily appreciated but the residual BPE less so (arrows).

Unexpected Malignancy

Traditionally, prior to the PSA era, in around 10% of TURPs carried out for clinically benign prostatic enlargement, histological examination revealed the presence of unsuspected malignancy. With PSA testing, this is a less frequent scenario, and an abnormal result will usually lead to investigations prior to any therapeutic prostate procedure. Even so, malignancy is sometimes identified in men with PSA within the normal reference range, then warranting postoperative evaluation. It is inherent that TURP and other procedures for BPE that remove tissue specimens do not sample the entire prostate, and particularly not the peripheral zone where malignancy more often arises (Figure 12.8); other treatment options may not provide any tissue for histological assessment. For evaluation of malignancy after prostate surgery, formal prostate biopsy is necessary and clinical practice is increasingly using diffusion-weighted MRI for identifying targets for biopsy as well as for radiological staging (see Chapter 13). After TURP, considerable imaging artifact limits the diagnostic value of MRI, and PSA may also be spuriously elevated for several weeks (Figure 12.9). Unless there is an imperative for more urgent investigation, representative imaging can be undertaken until around 6 months after surgery by which time the functional outcome will be evident and can be taken into account for management decisions.

Changes Over Time

Surgical debulking of the prostate does not halt the pathological process of BPE. The prostate continues to grow. This is particularly relevant to newer technologies whose long-term efficacy has not been established. In addition, age alters the neuromuscular function of the bladder, including development of overactivity, and nephrological function including decline in concentrating ability and onset of nocturnal polyuria. Older men may therefore develop LUTS at a varying interval after an apparently successful surgical procedure. It is important to investigate the causes of late recurrence of LUTS after prostate surgery as the causes may lie outside of the prostate.

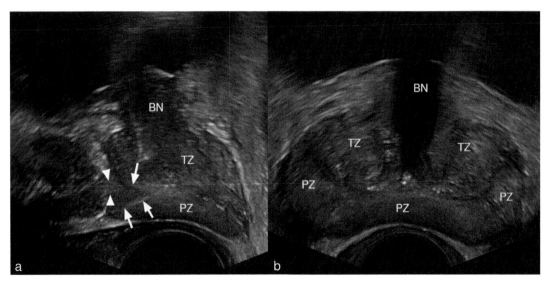

Figure 12.8 (a) Sagittal and (b) axial TRUS images of the prostate in a patient with BPE. The central zone is best shown on the sagittal image (a, arrows), with the seminal vesicle duct passing through it to form the ejaculatory duct (a, arrowheads). Transition zone (TZ), peripheral zone (PZ) and bladder neck (BN) are shown in each image.

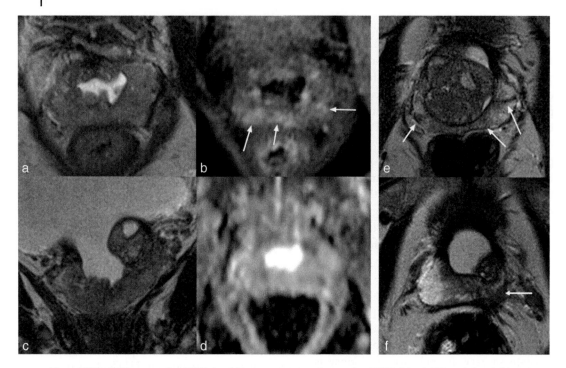

Figure 12.9 MRI images after TURP. (a–d) The same patient 1 year after TURP: (a) axial T2-weighted, (b) early dynamic post contrast, (c) coronal T2-weighted and (d) ADC map. The T2 signal in the peripheral zone is moderately reduced (a), and there is corresponding patchy enhancement (b, arrows) but not significantly restricted diffusion (d). Such appearances may last for years after TURP, with diffusion usually least affected. (e) T2 axial image from a different patient showing strands in the peripheral zone, a common appearance after TURP. (f) Tumour (arrow) on an MRI performed 2 years after TURP because of a rising prostate-specific antigen (PSA), and not sampled by the resection.

Re-operation after initial success is required in about 10% of men by 5–10 years, and may be necessary for residual or recurrent adenoma, urethral stricture or bladder neck stenosis [15, 44, 45]. Long-term follow-up studies after apparently successful surgery, however, indicate that recurrent symptoms more frequently indicate development of underactive bladder than obstruction [46].

Patients must be carefully counselled on outcomes of surgery for BPE guided by prior investigations; and this will significantly influence expectations by which surgical success may be judged.

References

1 Gratzke C, Bachmann A, Descazeaud A, *et al*. EAU guidelines on the assessment of non-neurogenic male lower urinary tract symptoms including benign prostatic obstruction. *Eur Urol*. 2015; 67(6): 1099–1109.

2 Kozminski MA, Wei JT, Nelson J, Kent DM. Baseline characteristics predict risk of progression and response to combined medical therapy for benign prostatic hyperplasia (BPH). *BJU Int*. 2015; 115(2): 308–316.

3 Yoshida T, Kinoshita H, Yoshida K, *et al*. Intravesical prostatic protrusion as a predicting factor for the adverse clinical outcome in patients with symptomatic

benign prostatic enlargement treated with dutasteride. *Urology.* 2016; 91: 154–157.

4 Park HY, Lee JY, Park SY, *et al.* Efficacy of alpha blocker treatment according to the degree of intravesical prostatic protrusion detected by transrectal ultrasonography in patients with benign prostatic hyperplasia. *Korean J Urol.* 2012; 53(2): 92–97.

5 Park JS, Lee HW, Lee SW, Moon HS, Park HY, Kim YT. Bladder wall thickness is associated with responsiveness of storage symptoms to alpha-blockers in men with lower urinary tract symptoms. *Korean J Urol.* 2012; 53(7): 487–491.

6 Ahmed AF. Sonographic parameters predicting the outcome of patients with lower urinary tract symptoms / benign prostatic hyperplasia treated with alpha1-adrenoreceptor antagonist. *Urology.* 2015; 88: 143–148.

7 Salah AS, Elsheikh MG. The impact of the bladder wall thickness on the outcome of the medical treatment using alpha-blocker of BPH patients with LUTS. *Aging Male.* 2015; 18(2): 89–92.

8 Cumpanas AA, Botoca M, Minciu R, Bucuras V. Intravesical prostatic protrusion can be a predicting factor for the treatment outcome in patients with lower urinary tract symptoms due to benign prostatic obstruction treated with tamsulosin. *Urology.* 2013; 81(4): 859–863.

9 Huang T, Qi J, Yu YJ, *et al.* Predictive value of resistive index, detrusor wall thickness and ultrasound estimated bladder weight regarding the outcome after transurethral prostatectomy for patients with lower urinary tract symptoms suggestive of benign prostatic obstruction. *Int J Urol.* 2012; 19(4): 343–350.

10 Hirayama K, Masui K, Hamada A, Shichiri Y, Masuzawa N, Hamada S. Evaluation of intravesical prostatic protrusion as a predictor of dutasteride-resistant lower urinary tract symptoms/benign prostatic enlargement with a high likelihood of surgical intervention. *Urology.* 2015; 86(3): 565–569.

11 Gravas S. Prostate volume as a risk factor for lower urinary tract symptoms: the quest continues. *Eur Urol.* 2016; 69(5): 892–893.

12 Cornu JN, Ahyai S, Bachmann A, *et al.* A Systematic review and meta-analysis of functional outcomes and complications following transurethral procedures for lower urinary tract symptoms resulting from benign prostatic obstruction: an update. *Eur Urol.* 2015; 67(6): 1066–1096.

13 Ahyai SA, Gilling P, Kaplan SA, *et al.* Meta-analysis of functional outcomes and complications following transurethral procedures for lower urinary tract symptoms resulting from benign prostatic enlargement. *Eur Urol.* 2010; 58(3): 384–397.

14 De NC, Tubaro A. Benign prostatic hyperplasia in 2014: innovations in medical and surgical treatment. *Nat Rev Urol.* 2015; 12(2): 76–78.

15 Madersbacher S, Marberger M. Is transurethral resection of the prostate still justified? *BJU Int.* 1999; 83(3): 227–237.

16 Elkoushy MA, Elshal AM, Elhilali MM. Holmium laser transurethral incision of the prostate: can prostate size predict the long-term outcome? *Can Urol Assoc J.* 2015; 9(7–8): 248–254.

17 Sivarajan G, Borofsky MS, Shah O, Lingeman JE, Lepor H. The role of minimally invasive surgical techniques in the management of large-gland benign prostatic hypertrophy. *Rev Urol.* 2015; 17(3): 140–149.

18 Li X, Pan JH, Liu QG, *et al.* Selective transurethral resection of the prostate combined with transurethral incision of the bladder neck for bladder outlet obstruction in patients with small volume benign prostate hyperplasia (BPH): a prospective randomized study. *PLoS One.* 2013; 8(5): e63227.

19 Gilling PJ, Wilson LC, King CJ, Westenberg AM, Frampton CM, Fraundorfer MR. Long-term results of a randomized trial comparing holmium laser enucleation of the prostate and transurethral resection of the prostate:

results at 7 years. *BJU Int.* 2012; 109(3): 408–411.

20 Hermanns T, Gross O, Kranzbuhler B, *et al.* Ablative efficiency of 532-nm laser vaporization compared to transurethral resection of the prostate: results from a prospective three-dimensional ultrasound volumetry study. *World J Urol.* 2014; 32(5): 1267–1274.

21 Geavlete B, Bulai C, Ene C, Checherita I, Geavlete P. Bipolar vaporization, resection, and enucleation versus open prostatectomy: optimal treatment alternatives in large prostate cases? *J Endourol.* 2015; 29(3): 323–331.

22 Rassweiler J, Teber D, Kuntz R, Hofmann R. Complications of transurethral resection of the prostate (TURP): incidence, management, and prevention. *Eur Urol.* 2006; 50(5): 969–979.

23 Chughtai B, Simma-Chiang V, Kaplan SA. Evaluation and management of post-transurethral resection of the prostate lower urinary tract symptoms. *Curr Urol Rep.* 2014; 15(9): 434.

24 Green W, Campain N, Peracha A, Ratan H, Walton T, Parkinson R. Very high residual volumes should not prevent transurethral resection of the prostate being offered to men presenting with urinary retention. *Scand J Urol.* 2014; 48(6): 549–553.

25 Aagaard J, Jonler M, Fuglsig S, Christensen LL, Jorgensen HS, Norgaard JP. Total transurethral resection versus minimal transurethral resection of the prostate: a 10-year follow-up study of urinary symptoms, uroflowmetry and residual volume. *Br J Urol.* 1994; 74(3): 333–336.

26 Muntener M, Aellig S, Kuettel R, Gehrlach C, Sulser T, Strebel RT. Sexual function after transurethral resection of the prostate (TURP): results of an independent prospective multicentre assessment of outcome. *Eur Urol.* 2007; 52(2): 510–515.

27 Marra G, Sturch P, Oderda M, Tabatabaei S, Muir G, Gontero P. Systematic review

of lower urinary tract symptoms/benign prostatic hyperplasia surgical treatments on men's ejaculatory function: time for a bespoke approach? *Int J Urol.* 2016; 23(1): 22–35.

28 Frieben RW, Lin HC, Hinh PP, Berardinelli F, Canfield SE, Wang R. The impact of minimally invasive surgeries for the treatment of symptomatic benign prostatic hyperplasia on male sexual function: a systematic review. *Asian J Androl.* 2010; 12(4): 500–508.

29 Gacci M, Ficarra V, Sebastianelli A, *et al.* Impact of medical treatments for male lower urinary tract symptoms due to benign prostatic hyperplasia on ejaculatory function: a systematic review and meta-analysis. *J Sex Med.* 2014; 11(6): 1554–1566.

30 Sturch P, Woo HH, McNicholas T, Muir G. Ejaculatory dysfunction after treatment for lower urinary tract symptoms: retrograde ejaculation or retrograde thinking? *BJU Int.* 2015; 115(2): 186–187.

31 Alloussi SH, Lang C, Eichel R, Alloussi S. Ejaculation-preserving transurethral resection of prostate and bladder neck: short- and long-term results of a new innovative resection technique. *J Endourol.* 2014; 28(1): 84–89.

32 Poulakis V, Ferakis N, Witzsch U, de Vries R, Becht E. Erectile dysfunction after transurethral prostatectomy for lower urinary tract symptoms: results from a center with over 500 patients. *Asian J Androl.* 2006; 8(1): 69–74.

33 Wasson JH, Reda DJ, Bruskewitz RC, Elinson J, Keller AM, Henderson WG. A comparison of transurethral surgery with watchful waiting for moderate symptoms of benign prostatic hyperplasia. The Veterans Affairs Cooperative Study Group on Transurethral Resection of the Prostate. *N Engl J Med.* 1995; 332(2): 75–79.

34 Favilla V, Cimino S, Salamone C, *et al.* Risk factors of sexual dysfunction after transurethral resection of the prostate (TURP): a 12 months

follow-up. *J Endocrinol Invest*. 2013; 36(11): 1094–1098.

35 Mishriki SF, Grimsley SJ, Lam T, Nabi G, Cohen NP. TURP and sex: patient and partner prospective 12 years follow-up study. *BJU Int*. 2012; 109(5): 745–750.

36 Soleimani M, Hosseini SY, Aliasgari M, Dadkhah F, Lashay A, Amini E. Erectile dysfunction after prostatectomy: an evaluation of the risk factors. *Scand J Urol Nephrol*. 2009; 43(4): 277–281.

37 Akman T, Binbay M, Tekinarslan E, *et al*. Effects of bipolar and monopolar transurethral resection of the prostate on urinary and erectile function: a prospective randomized comparative study. *BJU Int*. 2013; 111(1): 129–136.

38 Zong HT, Peng XX, Yang CC, Zhang Y. The impact of transurethral procedures for benign prostate hyperplasia on male sexual function: a meta-analysis. *J Androl*. 2012; 33(3): 427–434.

39 Bruyere F, Puichaud A, Pereira H, *et al*. Influence of photoselective vaporization of the prostate on sexual function: results of a prospective analysis of 149 patients with long-term follow-up. *Eur Urol*. 2010; 58(2): 207–211.

40 Kavoussi PK, Hermans MR. Maintenance of erectile function after photoselective vaporization of the prostate for obstructive benign prostatic hyperplasia. *J Sex Med*. 2008; 5(11): 2669–2671.

41 Bailey K, Abrams P, Blair PS, *et al*. Urodynamics for Prostate Surgery Trial; Randomised Evaluation of Assessment Methods (UPSTREAM) for diagnosis and management of bladder outlet obstruction in men: study protocol for a randomised controlled trial. *Trials*. 2015; 16: 567.

42 Madersbacher S, Klingler HC, Djavan B, *et al*. Is obstruction predictable by clinical evaluation in patients with lower urinary tract symptoms? *Br J Urol*. 1997; 80(1): 72–77.

43 Reynard JM, Yang Q, Donovan JL, *et al*. The ICS-'BPH' Study: uroflowmetry, lower urinary tract symptoms and bladder outlet obstruction. *Br J Urol*. 1998; 82(5): 619–623.

44 Roos NP, Wennberg JE, Malenka DJ, *et al*. Mortality and reoperation after open and transurethral resection of the prostate for benign prostatic hyperplasia. *N Engl J Med*. 1989; 320(17): 1120–1124.

45 Rieken M, Bachmann A, Shariat SF. Long-term follow-up data more than 5 years after surgical management of benign prostate obstruction: who stands the test of time? *Curr Opin Urol*. 2016; 26(1): 22–27.

46 Thomas AW, Cannon A, Bartlett E, Ellis-Jones J, Abrams P. The natural history of lower urinary tract dysfunction in men: minimum 10-year urodynamic followup of transurethral resection of prostate for bladder outlet obstruction. *J Urol*. 2005; 174(5): 1887–1891.

13

Imaging After Treatment of Prostate Cancer

Alex Kirkham

Introduction

In a man diagnosed with prostate cancer, the prostate may be removed, irradiated (with external beams or brachytherapy) or ablated. Focal therapy, by radiation and ablation, is becoming an accepted treatment in men with intermediate to low risk disease [1] and active surveillance a rational approach in many [2, 3]. Hormonal treatments can have significant effects on the appearance of the prostate [4].

The post-treatment imaging of men after treatment for prostate cancer has a common thread: with all modalities, recurrences can occur, and they usually have similar signal characteristics to tumour on pre-treatment scans [5]. However, the surroundings vary and we therefore arrange the chapter by modality, starting with radical prostatectomy.

Appearances After Radical Prostatectomy

The incidence of leaks after radical prostatectomy is around 9% on cystogram at 1 week, and they are associated with a lower rate of continence at 3 months (Figure 13.1) [6]. Computerised tomography (CT) cystography detects considerably more leaks (in up to one-third of patients in one study) [7], and shows that they are often small and contained, lying behind the urethra and bladder neck or extending into the prostatectomy bed although, less commonly, ileus and peritonitis can occur [8]. Magnetic resonance cystography is likely to have similar performance, although the additional complexity is probably not justified for routine use [9]. Transrectal ultrasound is an emerging alternative, with a good sensitivity, but some false positives resulting from peri-urethral fluid [10]. A leak indicates an incomplete anastomosis, which normally heals by secondary intention, associated with fibrosis and possibly a higher incidence of contracture [11], although this is debated [8], and the final rate of continence may be little lower [6]. If the leak is detected and the bladder drained, the normal course is gradual healing or obliteration of the contained leak cavity over weeks or months, although some irregularity may persist. The need for routine cystography is debated, however, with some limited evidence that omitting it from the postoperative pathway does not increase complications [12].

Lymphocoele occurs commonly after radical prostatectomy if a pelvic lymph node dissection is performed, but may still occur in 2.4–14% of patients who do not undergo lymphadenectomy [13, 14]. Lymphocoeles are seen as thin-walled, well-defined collections of close to water density on CT, or fluid signal on magnetic resonance imaging (MRI), and when small usually resolve spontaneously without symptoms (Figure 13.2).

Radiology and Follow-up of Urologic Surgery, First Edition. Edited by Christopher Woodhouse and Alex Kirkham.
© 2018 John Wiley & Sons Ltd. Published 2018 by John Wiley & Sons Ltd.

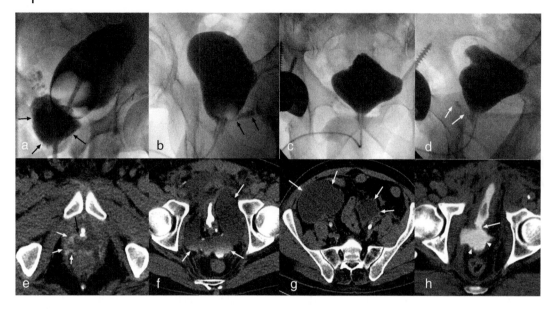

Figure 13.1 Anastomotic leaks after prostatectomy. (a,b) Large and small leaks at cystography 3 weeks after radical prostatectomy. (c) No leak is visible on the AP view. (d) Only on carefully turning the patient is a small anterior anastomotic leak visible. (e) Partial CT urogram in a different patient 1 week after prostatectomy shows a leak at the right side of the anastomosis (black arrow, with white arrows showing the extraperitoneal leak of contrast). (f,g) Extraperitoneal fluid tracking to upper pelvis (opacified posteriorly from the urogram) and lower abdomen in the same patient. (h) A CT cystogram in a different patient shows a large posterior anastomotic leak at 3 weeks (the arrow shows the defect).

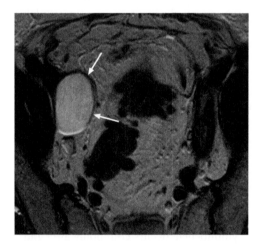

Figure 13.2 T2 axial image showing a lymphocoele 4 months after prostatectomy and lymph node dissection (arrows). Note that it is thin-walled, of fluid signal and distant from the vesico-urethral anastomosis.

When large they can occasionally cause pain or lower limb swelling and require treatment, usually by percutaneous drainage [15].

After prostatectomy the bladder neck has a funnelled appearance, and there are two main complications that may have imaging correlates: incontinence and obstruction from bladder neck contracture. There is some evidence that a longer length of external urethral sphincter on pre-operative MRI correlates with a reduced incidence of incontinence and one group has shown a similar association with both pre- and postoperative measurements of urethral length [16]. Others have not replicated this finding, but probably the most important association is with surgery for bladder neck contracture, which strongly increases the chance of incontinence [17]. Urethral hypermobility has been examined and probably does not strongly correlate with incontinence [18].

Symptomatic post-prostatectomy bladder neck contracture has an incidence of 8–16% [19, 20] and is usually suspected after a reduction in flow parameters, usually within 6 months and uncommon after 24 months [21]. Although often defined

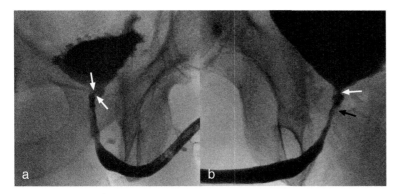

Figure 13.3 Two examples of bladder neck contractures (performed on an ascending urethrogram as part of a video-urodynamics study). (a) A patient 2 years after radical prostatectomy. There is a short, tight stricture at the bladder neck (arrows), difficult to appreciate on any of the fluoroscopy views at the time (this is the best image). The retrograde urethral leak point pressure was low (indicating sphincter weakness) but the urethral pressure profile was high (>100 cm water). This is because the 8 Fr pressure profile catheter was only just admitted into the bladder: the stricture then caused an artefactually high 'sphincter' pressure at the neck. (b) A different patient who has undergone high intensity focused ultrasound (HIFU) and radiotherapy for prostate cancer. The bladder neck stricture (white arrow) was causing obstructed voiding; the prostatic cavity below is short and irregular. The veru (black arrow) is still seen but not obstructing.

as the inability to pass a cystoscope past the bladder neck [22], it can be confirmed most reliably on video-urodynamics, when the anatomical abnormality is shown on imaging (Figure 13.3) and obstruction confirmed by the pressure–flow relationship. This test is also very useful in the context of incontinence, to distinguish several different possible causes: reduced compliance, detrusor overactivity or sphincter weakness [23]. The latter can be difficult to show with conventional Valsalva and cough provocation, with some men who have clear sphincter weakness not leaking during the test [24], and either urethral pressure profilometry [25] or retrograde leak point pressure measurement (which is simpler and requires less specialist equipment) [26] are likely to be more accurate.

it shows restriction, high signal on long b sequences and bright early enhancement, as on a primary diagnostic scan (Figure 13.4). It most commonly occurs close to the anastomosis, but can be seen anywhere in the surgical bed and at the site of transection of vas and vesicle [29]. A recent paper assessed the performance of: (i) T2, (ii) T2 and diffusion, (iii) T2 and dynamically enhanced and (iv) T2, diffusion and enhanced sequences. The best results were obtained with contrast and T2 sequences, and adding diffusion sequences had little impact: sensitivity was 77–82% and specificity 83–87% [30]. Others have confirmed that enhancement is essential (and most sensitive), but found diffusion imaging of paramount importance in the case of enhancement from surrounding structures (in particular veins) [31].

Residual Tumour After Radical Prostatectomy

On T2 sequences residual tumour can appear relatively hyperintense to the surrounding post-surgical fibrosis or muscle [27, 28] but on diffusion and enhanced sequences

The Prostate After Ablative Therapies

Although focal therapy is becoming an established method for treating localised prostate cancer [32], most of the published experience of prostate ablation comes from

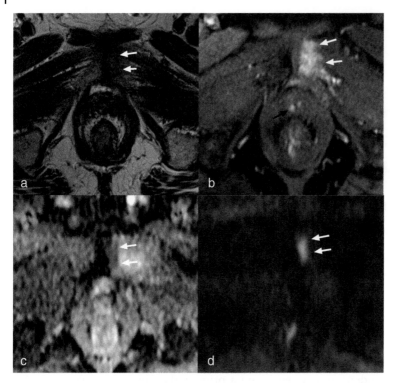

Figure 13.4 Residual tumour on MRI 1.5 years after prostatectomy in a man with prostate-specific antigen (PSA) level of 4. (a) The T2 sequence shows no convincing abnormality in the region of the anastomosis, but subtle slightly asymmetrically low signal in the left pubic bone (arrows). (b) An early dynamically enhanced image and shows a tiny focus of residual tumour at the anastomosis (black arrow) as well as enhancement in the L pubic bone. (c,d) An ADC map and b2000 diffusion-weighted image; the tumour is too small to be seen (the enhanced images are more sensitive for small volumes) but the metastasis in the bone is well shown (arrows).

studies of treatment of the whole prostate. We might broadly split the techniques into heating, cooling and irradiation. The last is not really the subject of this book, but will be addressed briefly in the context of brachytherapy. We predominantly describe the ablative technologies and, as well as describing the expected appearances, we make the case for imaging both early after treatment and later to detect residual tumour.

Early Appearances

We know that early after whole gland ablation the prostate swells, with a volume increase of around 50% in the first 2 weeks [33], and we have observed similar increases in volume in the treated quadrant of the prostate after focal therapy. All ablation modalities aim to produce confluent necrosis that covers the tumour, while minimising morbidity from damage to adjacent structures (in particular the external sphincter and cavernosal nerves) [34]. While there are changes in the diffusion characteristics of treated prostate [35], techniques assessing perfusion are likely to have a higher spatial resolution for the assessment of necrosis, and while contrast ultrasound (US) has been used to assess perfusion after high intensity focused US (HIFU) [36], enhanced MRI allows a standardised technique and comparison with pre-operative imaging showing the tumour [36].

The technique for early scans can be similar to the European Society for Urological

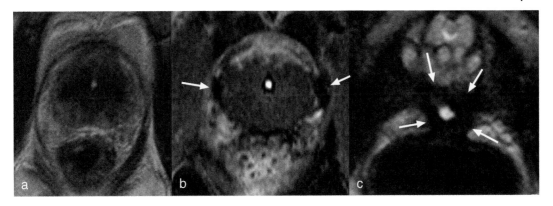

Figure 13.5 Appearances after whole gland HIFU. (a,b) T2 and late enhanced sequences 1 week after treatment. There is patchy T2 change, but only the enhanced images shows the margins of the necrosis well (and a little lateral extra prostatic necrosis too;b, arrows). (c) At 6 months there is a small amount of uniformly low T2 signal material in the position of the prostate (arrows), with the urethra passing through the middle. Biopsy showed no evidence of residual tumour.

Radiology (ESUR) guidelines for diagnostic MRI [37], with diffusion scans omitted. Dynamically enhanced sequences are adequate but standard spin echo pre- and post-contrast T1 images are of slightly higher resolution and may be substituted. The best time for scanning to show the treated volume is probably the first week: we know that prostate volume after whole gland treatment can shrink by up to 50% in the first month [38].

The T2 appearances are heterogeneous and cannot be used to assess necrosis (Figure 13.5). After contrast, complete ablation usually results in a homogenous, non-enhancing focus (subtracted images can be useful to allow for post-treatment haemorrhage), although the margins may be indistinct, with enhancing strands, and after HIFU an enhancing, usually continuous, rim measuring 2–8 mm in diameter [33].

An early scan has the potential to provide feedback to the operator about the accuracy and completeness of the ablation, and potentially to predict early complications. How accurately does non-perfusion predict necrosis? In cryotherapy, early studies suggested that if the non-enhancing zone covered the position of the tumour, recurrence was unlikely [39], but subsequent analyses have found residual viable tumour inside the margins of apparently complete non-enhancement [40]. A study using a prototype transurethral HIFU device in dogs and assessing necrosis in prostatectomy specimens suggested that non-enhancement did indeed imply complete necrosis [41], but the accuracy probably depends on both the ablative technology used and the MRI technique employed.

Early Complications

Aside from necrosis extending outside the intended volume (whether in whole gland or focal treatments), the main early complication of ablation is fistulation, either anteriorly into the symphisis (Figure 13.6) [42] or posteriorly into the rectum (Figure 13.7) [43]. Necrosis extending outside the prostate is common after primary ablation, and usually of no consequence even if it involves a significant part of the rectal muscularis, but after radiotherapy (in particular, brachytherapy) is much more likely to cause fistulation, presenting weeks to months after the treatment [43, 44]. In patients undergoing MRI for suspected rectal fistulation, the finding of air within the prostate is suggestive, and the tract can often be seen on T2, short T1 inversion recovery (STIR) and post-contrast sequences.

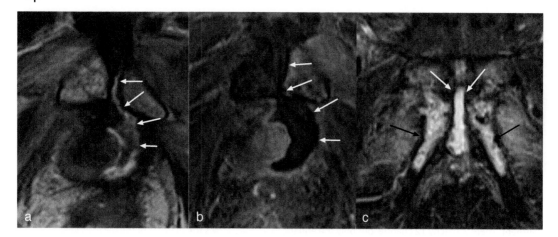

Figure 13.6 Anterior fistulation. (a,b) T2 and post-contrast images of a patient who presented with suprapubic pain 5 months after HIFU. Fluid (high signal on T2, low on the enhanced image) is tracking into the symphisis (arrows). (c) STIR image showing an anterior fistula in a different patient who underwent salvage HIFU for recurrent tumour after radiotherapy: the white arrows show fluid in the symphysis and the black arrows chronic radiation-induced osteonecrosis in the pubic bones.

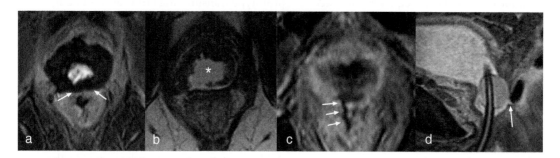

Figure 13.7 Posterior fistulation. (a,b) Post-contrast and T2-weighted images 3 months after salvage HIFU for recurrent prostate cancer after radiotherapy. Note the rectal wall necrosis (not quite involving the mucosa: arrows). In a patient who had not undergone radiotherapy this would be very unlikely to develop into a fistula. (c,d) Images at 7 months (c, axial T1, early after contrast; d, sagittal STIR) showing the established fistula.

Appearances at 2–5 Months

The appearances at 2–5 months are variable: resorption of necrotic tissue is taking place (and is usually complete at 6 months if there has not been previous radiotherapy) and the enhancing rim persists (and in some cases may be seen as a double rim) [33]. This makes it difficult to assess the prostate for residual tumour, and we usually wait until 6 months (or 1 year after radiotherapy) to do so.

Appearances at 6 Months: Assessing Residual and Recurrent Tumour

At 6 months, the ablated prostate is usually replaced by fibrosis: low in T2 signal and showing delayed, moderate enhancement (as elsewhere in the body) [45]. After focal therapy we have observed inflammatory-type signal change (mildly reduced T2 signal and moderately prominent enhancement) in the adjacent (and even contralateral) prostate that can persist for several years (Figure 13.8).

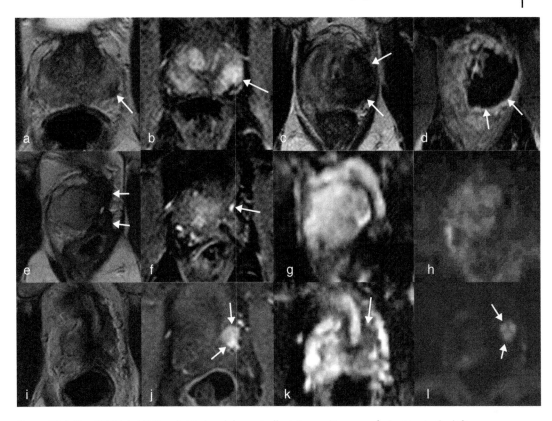

Figure 13.8 Focal HIFU. (a,b) T2-weighted and dynamically enhanced images of a tumour in the left posterolateral peripheral zone (arrow). (c,d) T2 and post-contrast images 1 week after treatment; only the post-contrast image defines the necrosis well (arrows). (e–h) T2-weighted, dynamically enhanced, ADC map and diffusion-weighted (b1400) images 2 years later, after one further HIFU treatment for radiological recurrence. A small focus of recurrent tumour is seen on the enhanced image (arrows) but not on the T2 or diffusion-weighted sequences. Biopsy at this point was negative. (i–l) The same sequences 15 months later: the tumour is easily seen on enhanced and diffusion-weighted images (arrows) but remains hard to distinguish from post-HIFU fibrosis on the T2 sequence.

The fibrosis can make residual low T2 signal tumour difficult to see, and it is important to use a multiparametric protocol including diffusion and enhanced sequences [37]. The ADC map of the diffusion sequences can also be confusing, because fibrosis can appear as an absence of signal, and the long b sequence (showing high signal in relatively cellular tumour) [46] is particularly important. Tumour can be very conspicuous early after contrast because of the late, mild enhancement of fibrosis, but inflammation and residual prostate can enhance brightly too, so that contrast may be most sensitive and diffusion most specific: in one study diffusion images had a sensitivity of 66% and specificity of 76%, with dynamically enhanced sequences showing a sensitivity of 83% and specificity 66% (it is likely that a truly multisequence approach will be most successful) [47]. One group found a sensitivity of 75% and a specificity of 76% for the detection of tumour using contrast after whole gland HIFU [48], similar in performance to prostate-specific antigen (PSA) criteria (sensitivity of 78% and specificity of 79% for PSA nadir +1.2 ng/L in the whole gland HIFU registry [49]. Whether MRI will have a better performance than PSA criteria in the era of focal therapy is difficult to say, but it is likely to have an important role in follow-up for the detection of residual or recurrent tumour: repeat biopsies are invasive and potentially morbid, and can also miss tumours unless targeted to MRI findings [50]. A recent study comparing MRI (in most cases with a protocol of T2 and dynamically enhanced sequences) with PSA for the detection of recurrence at biopsy showed that in many cases MRI was more accurate, with a higher area under the ROC curve [51].

After radiotherapy (both external beam and brachytherapy), the prostate is generally smaller, with a loss of T2 signal and zonal differentiation [52]. This means that recurrent tumours are relatively hard to see on T2 sequences, but conspicuous on both enhanced and diffusion-weighted images, even if the there are low dose brachytherapy seeds. The figures for the detection of significant tumour are similar to those in the untreated prostate [53, 54].

Nuclear Medicine Studies

Conventional fluorodeoxyglucose positron emission tomography (FDG PET) is considerably less sensitive than MRI for the detection of tumour both after radical prostatectomy and ablation. Choline-based agents are more sensitive, but cannot match the sensitivity of MRI in patients with PSA <1 ng/mL [55]; in a recent study of MRI the performance for the detection of local recurrence was excellent with a median PSA of 0.43 ng/mL [30]. Prostate specific membrane antigen-based agents are likely even better, but as yet unproven [56]. The combination of detection and localisation with multiparametric MRI is likely to remain the gold standard for some time.

A Schedule for Follow-up

PSA remains the primary method for the detection of residual tumour after prostatectomy and whole gland ablation, so that it is impossible to give a widely applicable schedule for the use of imaging (in particular, MRI). However, in the era of focal therapy – where PSA is potentially harder to interpret – this balance may shift, and the routine use of MRI may become more widespread [51].

References

1 Polascik TJ. *Imaging and Focal Therapy of Early Prostate Cancer*. Springer Science & Business Media; 2012: 1.
2 Polascik TJ, Mouraviev V. Focal therapy for prostate cancer. *Curr Opin Urol*. 2008; 18(3): 269–274.
3 Parker C. Active surveillance: towards a new paradigm in the management of early prostate cancer. *Lancet Oncol*. 2004; 5(2): 101–106.
4 Groenendaal G, van Vulpen M, Pereboom SR, *et al.* Radiotherapy and oncology. *Radiother Oncol*. 2012; 103(2): 233–238.
5 Rouvière O, Vitry T, Lyonnet D. Imaging of prostate cancer local recurrences: why and how? *Eur Radiol*. 2009; 20(5): 1254–1266.
6 Patil N, Krane L, Javed K, Williams T, Bhandari M, Menon M. Evaluating and grading cystographic leakage: correlation with clinical outcomes in patients undergoing robotic prostatectomy. *BJU Int*. 2009; 103(8): 1108–1110.
7 Han KS, Choi HJ, Jung DC, *et al.* A prospective evaluation of conventional cystography for detection of urine leakage at the vesicourethral anastomosis site after radical prostatectomy based on computed tomography. *Clin Radiol*. 2011; 66(3): 251–256.
8 Tyritzis SI, Katafigiotis I, Constantinides CA. All you need to know about urethrovesical anastomotic urinary leakage following radical prostatectomy. *J Urol*. 2012; 188(2): 369–376.
9 Tonolini M, Villa F, Bianco R. Multidetector CT imaging of post-robot-assisted laparoscopic radical prostatectomy

complications. *Insights Imaging*. 2013; 4(5): 711–721.

10 Eggert T, Palisaar J, Metz P, Noldus J. Assessing the vesico-urethral anastomosis after radical retropubic prostatectomy: transrectal ultrasonography can replace cystography. *BJU Int*. 2007; 100(6): 1268–1271.

11 Webb DR, Sethi K, Gee K. An analysis of the causes of bladder neck contracture after open and robot-assisted laparoscopic radical prostatectomy. *BJU Int*. 2009; 103(7): 957–963.

12 Guru KA, Seereiter PJ, Sfakianos JP, Hutson AD, Mohler JL. Is a cystogram necessary after robot-assisted radical prostatectomy? *Urol Oncol*. 2007; 25(6): 465–467.

13 Khoder WY, Trottmann M, Buchner A, *et al.* Risk factors for pelvic lymphoceles post-radical prostatectomy. *Int J Urol*. 2011; 18: 638–643.

14 Augustin H, Hammerer P, Graefen M, *et al.* Intraoperative and perioperative morbidity of contemporary radical retropubic prostatectomy in a consecutive series of 1243 patients: results of a single center between 1999 and 2002. *Eur Urol*. 2003; 43(2): 113–118.

15 Pepper RJ, Pati J, Kaisary AV. The incidence and treatment of lymphoceles after radical retropubic prostatectomy. *BJU Int*. 2005; 95(6): 772–775.

16 Coakley FV, Eberhardt S, Kattan MW, Wei DC, Scardino PT, Hricak H. Urinary continence after radical retropubic prostatectomy: relationship with membranous urethral length on preoperative endorectal magnetic resonance imaging. *J Urol*. 2002; 168(3): 1032–1035.

17 Kordan Y, Alkibay T, Sozen S, *et al.* Is there an impact of postoperative urethral and periurethral anatomical features in post-radical retropubic prostatectomy incontinence? *Urol Int*. 2007; 78(3): 208–213.

18 Suskind AM, DeLancey JOL, Hussain HK, Montgomery JS, Latini JM, Cameron AP. Dynamic MRI evaluation of urethral

hypermobility post-radical prostatectomy. *Neurourol Urodynam*. 2013; 33(3): 312–315.

19 Elliott S, Meng M, Elkin E, Mcaninch J, Duchane J, Carroll P. Incidence of urethral stricture after primary treatment for prostate cancer: data from CaPSURE. *J Urol*. 2007; 178(2): 529–534.

20 Stanford JL, Feng Z, Hamilton AS, *et al.* Urinary and sexual function after radical prostatectomy for clinically localized prostate cancer: the Prostate Cancer Outcomes Study. *JAMA*. 2000; 283(3): 354–360.

21 Elliott DS, Boone TB. Combined stent and artificial urinary sphincter for management of severe recurrent bladder neck contracture and stress incontinence after prostatectomy: a long-term evaluation. *J Urol*. 2001; 165(2): 413–415.

22 Brede C, Angermeier K, Wood H. Radical prostatectomycontinence outcomes after treatment of recalcitrant postprostatectomy bladder neck contracture and review of the literature. *Urology*. 2014; 83(3): 648–652.

23 Chao R, Mayo ME. Incontinence after radical prostatectomy: detrusor or sphincter causes. *J Urol*. 1995; 154(1): 16–18.

24 Weissbart SJ, Coutinho K, Chughtai B, Sandhu JS. Characteristics and outcomes of men who fail to leak on intubated urodynamics prior to artificial urinary sphincter placement. *Can J Urol*. 2014; 21(6): 7560–7564.

25 Dubbelman YD, Bosch JLHR. Urethral sphincter function before and after radical prostatectomy: systematic review of the prognostic value of various assessment techniques. *Neurourol Urodynam*. 2013; 32(7): 957–963.

26 Comiter CV, Sullivan MP, Yalla SV. Correlation among maximal urethral closure pressure, retrograde leak point pressure, and abdominal leak point pressure in men with postprostatectomy stress incontinence. *Urology*. 2003; 62(1): 75–78.

27 Panebianco V, Barchetti F, Grompone MD, *et al.* Magnetic resonance imaging

for localization of prostate cancer in the setting of biochemical recurrence. *Urol Oncol*. 2016; 34(7):1–8.

28 Vargas HA, Wassberg C, Akin O, Hricak H. MR Imaging of treated prostate cancer. *Radiology*. 2012; 262(1): 26–42.

29 Sella T, Schwartz LH, Swindle PW, *et al*. Suspected local recurrence after radical prostatectomy: endorectal coil MR imaging. *Radiology*. 2004; 231(2): 379–385.

30 Kitajima K, Hartman RP, Froemming AT, Hagen CE, Takahashi N, Kawashima A. Detection of local recurrence of prostate cancer after radical prostatectomy using endorectal coil MRI at 3 T: addition of DWI and dynamic contrast enhancement to T2-weighted MRI. *Am J Roentgenol*. 2015; 205(4): 807–816.

31 Panebianco V, Barchetti F, Sciarra A, *et al*. Prostate cancer recurrence after radical prostatectomy: the role of 3-T diffusion imaging in multi-parametric magnetic resonance imaging. *Eur Radiol*. 2013; 23(6): 1745–1752.

32 Valerio M, Ahmed HU, Emberton M, *et al*. The role of focal therapy in the management of localised prostate cancer: a systematic review. *Eur Urol*. 2014; 66(4): 732–751.

33 Kirkham APS, Emberton M, Hoh IM, Illing RO, Freeman AA, Allen C. MR imaging of prostate after treatment with high-intensity focused ultrasound. *Radiology*. 2008; 246(3): 833–844.

34 Ahmed HU, Dickinson L, Charman S, *et al*. Focal ablation targeted to the index lesion in multifocal localised prostate cancer: a prospective development study. *Eur Urol*. 2015; 68(6): 1–10.

35 Chen J, Daniel BL, Diederich CJ, *et al*. Monitoring prostate thermal therapy with diffusion-weighted MRI. *Magn Reson Med*. 2008; 59(6): 1365–1372.

36 Rouvière O, Glas L, Girouin N, *et al*. Prostate cancer ablation with transrectal high-intensity focused ultrasound: assessment of tissue destruction with contrast-enhanced US. *Radiology*. 2011; 259(2): 583–591.

37 Weinreb JC, Barentsz JO, Choyke PL, *et al*. PI-RADS prostate imaging: reporting and data system: 2015, Version 2. *Eur Urol*. 2016; 69(1): 16–40.

38 Rouviere O, Souchon R, Salomir R, Gelet A, Chapelon J, Lyonnet D. Transrectal high-intensity focused ultrasound ablation of prostate cancer: effective treatment requiring accurate imaging. *Eur J Radiol*. 2007; 63(3): 317–327.

39 Vellet AD, Saliken J, Donnelly B, *et al*. Prostatic cryosurgery: use of MR imaging in evaluation of success and technical modifications. *Radiology*. 1997; 203(3): 653–659.

40 Donnelly SE, Donnelly BJ, Saliken JC, Raber EL, Vellet AD. Prostate cancer: gadolinium-enhanced MR imaging at 3 weeks compared with needle biopsy at 6 months after cryoablation. *Radiology*. 2004; 232: 830–833.

41 Boyes A, Tang K, Yaffe M, Sugar L, Chopra R, Bronskill M. Prostate tissue analysis immediately following magnetic resonance imaging guided transurethral ultrasound thermal therapy. *J Urol*. 2007; 178(3): 1080–1085.

42 Bugeja S, Andrich DE, Mundy AR. Fistulation into the pubic symphysis after treatment of prostate cancer: an important and surgically correctable complication. *J Urol*. 2016; 195(2): 391–398.

43 Ahmed HU, Ishaq A, Zacharakis E, *et al*. Rectal fistulae after salvage high-intensity focused ultrasound for recurrent prostate cancer after combined brachytherapy and external beam radiotherapy. *BJU Int*. 2009; 103(3): 321–323.

44 Sanchez A, Rodríguez D, Cheng J-S, McGovern FJ, Tabatabaei S. Prostatic diseases and male voiding dysfunction prostato-symphyseal fistula after photoselective vaporization of the prostate: case series and literature review of a rare complication. *Urology*. 2015; 85(1): 172–177.

45 Lucht REA, Delorme S, Hei J, *et al.* Classification of signal-time curves obtained by dynamic magnetic resonance mammography: statistical comparison of quantitative methods. *Invest Radiol.* 2005; 40(7): 442–447.

46 Rosenkrantz AB, Hindman N, Lim RP, *et al.* Diffusion-weighted imaging of the prostate: comparison of b1000 and b2000 image sets for index lesion detection. *J Magn Reson Imaging.* 2013; 38(3): 694–700.

47 Kim CK, Park BK, Lee HM, Kim SS, Kim E. MRI techniques for prediction of local tumor progression after high-intensity focused ultrasonic ablation of prostate cancer. *Am J Roentgenol.* 2008; 190(5): 1180–1186.

48 Punwani S, Emberton M, Walkden M, *et al.* Prostatic cancer surveillance following whole-gland high-intensity focused ultrasound: comparison of MRI and prostate-specific antigen for detection of residual or recurrent disease. *Br J Radiol.* 2012; 85(1014): 720–728.

49 Blana A, Brown SCW, Chaussy C, *et al.* High-intensity focused ultrasound for prostate cancer: comparative definitions of biochemical failure. *BJU Int.* 2009; 104(8): 1058–1062.

50 Rouvière O, Girouin N, Glas L, *et al.* Prostate cancer transrectal HIFU ablation: detection of local recurrences using T2-weighted and dynamic contrast-enhanced MRI. *Eur Radiol.* 2009; 20(1): 48–55.

51 Dickinson L, Ahmed HU, Hindley RG, *et al.* Prostate-specific antigen vs. magnetic resonance imaging parameters for assessing oncological outcomes after high intensity-focused ultrasound focal therapy for localized prostate cancer. *Urol Oncol.* 2017; 35(1): 30.

52 De Visschere PJL, Vargas HA, Ost P, De Meerleer GO, Villeirs GM. Imaging treated prostate cancer. *Abdom Imaging.* 2013; 38(6): 1431–1446.

53 Arumainayagam N, Kumaar S, Ahmed HU, *et al.* Accuracy of multiparametric magnetic resonance imaging in detecting recurrent prostate cancer after radiotherapy. *BJU Int.* 2010; 106(7): 991–997.

54 Fütterer JJ, Briganti A, De Visschere P, *et al.* Can clinically significant prostate cancer be detected with multiparametric magnetic resonance imaging? A systematic review of the literature. *Eur Urol.* 2015; 68(6): 1045–1053.

55 Evangelista L, Cimitan M, Hodolič M, Baseric T, Fettich J, Borsatti E. The ability of 18F-choline PET/CT to identify local recurrence of prostate cancer. *Abdom Imaging.* 2015; 40(8): 3230–3237.

56 Rowe SP, Gorin MA, Allaf ME, *et al.* PET imaging of prostate-specific membrane antigen in prostate cancer: current state of the art and future challenges. *Prostate Cancer Prostatic Dis.* 2016; 19(3): 223–230.

14

Urethroplasty

Simon Bugeja, Clare Allen and Daniella E. Andrich

Introduction

The management of urethral strictures has evolved over the years. The simplest forms of intervention remain urethral dilatation and optical urethrotomy in the hope that healing by secondary intention will occur before further scarring [1]. The 'curative' rate is only around 60% and this only in short strictures of the bulbar urethra [2]. The long-term success rate and cost effectiveness decrease even further with subsequent attempts at endoscopic intervention [3]. Therefore, in longer penile and bulbar strictures, congenital strictures of the penile urethra (hypospadias) and post-traumatic strictures, the only curative treatment option is urethroplasty.

Contrast imaging (retrograde and antegrade urethrography) forms an important part of the pre-operative evaluation of urethral strictures but is also the most common radiological investigation used in postoperative follow-up. Fifty-one per cent of articles in a systematic review of the literature used urethrography as a primary diagnostic tool for stricture recurrence [4]. Urethrography is performed in the early postoperative period in order to evaluate healing prior to catheter removal (pericatheter urethrogram, PUG) [5] and at various intervals thereafter in order to detect stricture recurrence.

Pericatheter Urethrogram

A urethral catheter is routinely used after any urethroplasty in order to stent the repair until healed. A PUG objectively confirms healing by the absence of extravasation of contrast [6]. A 6-Fr tube is passed alongside the indwelling urethral catheter and 10–30 mL water-soluble contrast gently injected under fluoroscopy, holding the penis on traction to obtain lateral views of the urethra at the site of the urethroplasty. The ideal time interval before catheter removal remains unknown but is generally between 1 and 3 weeks [7, 8]. In our practice, we perform PUG at 2 weeks on all patients having routine penile or bulbar urethroplasty, 3 weeks following bulbo-prostatic anastomotic (BPA) or urorectal fistula repair and at 6 weeks after urethral reconstruction if the patient has had radiotherapy. If extravasation is detected, the catheter is left in situ for another week and the procedure repeated (Figure 14.1) at which time 85% of leaks have resolved.

Prolonged radiological leak, particularly after penile urethroplasty, may indicate development of a urethro-cutaneous fistula, usually related to an infected suture or insufficient dartos interposition with wound breakdown. Once the catheter is seen through the suture line, such a defect will

Radiology and Follow-up of Urologic Surgery, First Edition. Edited by Christopher Woodhouse and Alex Kirkham.
© 2018 John Wiley & Sons Ltd. Published 2018 by John Wiley & Sons Ltd.

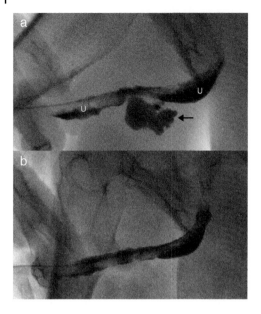

Figure 14.1 (a) Pericatheter urethrogram 2 weeks after a single stage penile urethroplasty showing a large contrast leak from the suture line ventrally (arrow). (b) One week later the leak has resolved completely and the catheter can be removed.

never heal spontaneously and the catheter is best removed with a view to repair of a mature fistula a few months later. However, particularly after anastomotic repairs of the bulbar urethra, a small anastomotic leak can create a small contained peri-urethral cavity, and is usually of no clinical consequence (Figure 14.2).

Ascending and Descending Urethrography

Complete assessment of stricture length, calibre and location is only achieved by a combined ascending (retrograde) and descending (antegrade or voiding) urethrogram.

The aim of the ascending study is to visualise the distal end and assess the length and diameter of the stricture. Radio-opaque contrast is injected urethrally in order to distend and delineate the penile and bulbar urethra usually up to the external urethral sphincter.

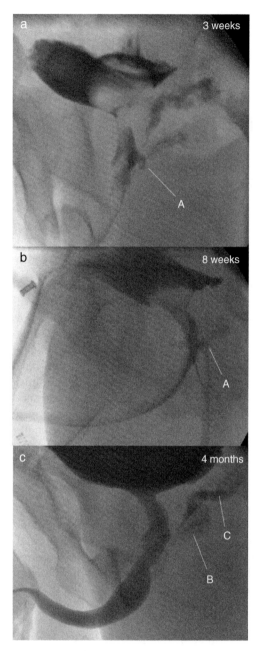

Figure 14.2 Pericatheter urethrogram sequence after a bulbo-prostatic anastomotic urethroplasty. (a) At 3 weeks a small leak is visible at the anastomotic site (A) which is still visible at 8 weeks (b) at which time the catheter was removed. (c) At 4 months there is no stricture recurrence. Note intra-prostatic reflux of contrast (B) and up the left seminal vesicle (C) which might be mistaken for a leak.

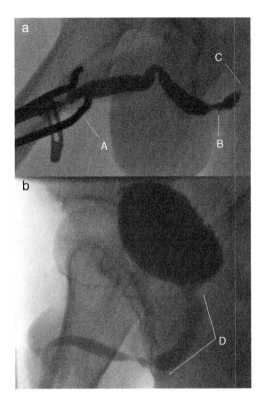

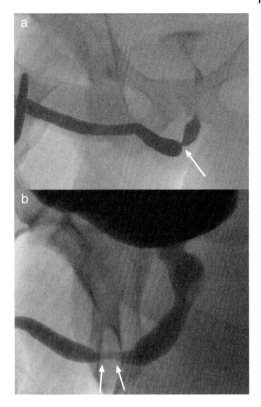

Figure 14.3 (a) Retrograde urethrogram (RUG) using Knutson's clamp (A) distending the entire penile and bulbar urethra. There is a mid-bulbar stricture (B) and contrast fails to distend the external sphincter complex (C). (b) Voiding study in the same patient showing prestenotic dilatation of the prostatic and proximal bulbar urethra (D) indicating obstruction to flow. Note how the stricture is better seen on the more lateral view.

Figure 14.4 Bulbar stricture (arrow) after anastomotic urethroplasty. (a) Stricture is foreshortened. (b) True stricture length is now clear on lateral view on voiding study.

When the patient is able to relax the external urethral sphincter, the prostatic urethra and bladder can also be visualised (Figure 14.3).

Serial fluoroscopic images are obtained whilst the penis is held on traction to obtain lateral views of the urethra to avoid foreshortening of the stricture (Figure 14.4). One should avoid undue urethral filling pressure to prevent urethral over-distension which may lead to urothelial rupture and extravasation. We use a Knutson's clamp to create an adequate seal of the glandular urethra which causes less urethral trauma and patient discomfort than a partially inflated Foley catheter balloon in the navicular fossa.

A voiding study provides a dynamic evaluation of a urethral stricture and will delineate the proximal end of the stricture; the prostatic and bulbar urethra proximal to the stricture will distend, confirming that the stricture is causing outflow obstruction (Figure 14.3b). In obliterative strictures, 250 mL contrast is instilled into the bladder via the suprapubic catheter. The patient is asked to relax and 'to imagine to void', so that the bladder neck sphincter can relax, allowing contrast to enter the prostatic urethra down to the proximal end of the obliterative stricture (Figure 14.5a).

Radiological Appearance After Different Types of Urethroplasty

The radiological appearance of the urethra after urethroplasty will vary according to the

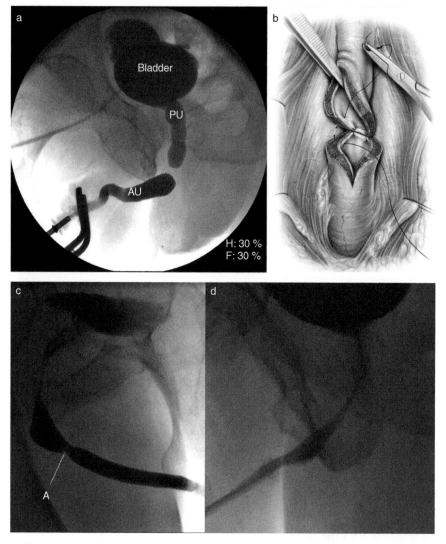

Figure 14.5 (a) Ascending and descending (via suprapubic tube) urethrogram showing the defect and urethral tissue loss of a fall-astride mid-bulbar segment. AU, anterior urethra; PU, posterior urethra. (b) Spatulated end-to-end anastomosis after stricture excision. Source: Mundy 2005 [10]. Reproduced with permission of John Wiley and Sons. (c) Retrograde and antegrade postoperative urethrogram showing that the site of anastomotic repair (A) is slightly reduced in calibre, but does not cause distension of the prostatic and proximal bulbar urethra (d); therefore the relative recurrent stricture is not flow-significant and can be followed-up conservatively.

type of procedure performed which in turn is dependent on stricture location, aetiology, length and previous intervention [9].

Traumatic Strictures

In traumatic strictures, a urethral segment has been crushed by a severe force (fall astride on to perineum, or pelvic fracture-related urethral crush or laceration from a pelvic bone spike or complete disruption of the urethra). This high energy impact causes cell death. The dead urethral spongiosal tissue is absorbed during the healing process, eventually leading to transmural fibrosis or loss of the entire urethral segment affected.

As a principle, traumatic urethral strictures are repaired by excision and end-to-end anastomosis (i.e. suturing the healthy ends together). Depending on the length and location of the urethral loss, this can be technically more or less challenging. Spatulating the urethral ends of the anastomosis produces an oblique suture line with less chance of contracting during the healing process (Figure 14.5) [10]. The site can be often identified as a diamond-shaped area on follow-up urethrogram (Figure 14.6).

Idiopathic Bulbar Strictures

In idiopathic bulbar strictures, the spongiofibrosis is remarkably superficial. Therefore an anastomotic technique is possible where the spongiofibrosis is short and can be excised, preserving the healthy part of the bulbar corpus spongiosum and bulbar arteries (Figure 14.7) [11]. This non-transecting approach can be augmented with buccal mucosal graft in longer strictures if necessary [12]. In long bulbar strictures without a particularly tight segment, oral mucosal graft augmentation is used on its own. The graft can be placed dorsally (our preference in most cases) or ventrally [13]. The characteristic radiological appearance after graft augmentation bulbar urethroplasty is a 'wider than normal' segment where the patch has been placed and which sometimes appears irregular. Most men will have some degree of post-micturition dribbling and reduced force of ejaculation, as inevitably a few drops are trapped in the grafted urethral segment. Contrast may be seen to pool in the reconstructed urethral segment on a post-void image in these patients (Figure 14.8c).

Penile Urethroplasty

Penile urethral strictures cannot be managed by excision and primary anastomosis because of the risk of penile shortening and chordee. There are different surgical techniques used for the different aetiologies.

For example, patients who have had proximal hypospadias repair in childhood and develop recurrent strictures later in life, have in fact a stenosed old foreskin flap tube which has become ischaemic over the years. Hence, the entire hypospadias repair segment often has to be replaced. In such cases, oral mucosal grafts are used to substitute (re-build) a new urethral plate (Figure 14.9a). This has to be carried out in two operations, usually 6 months apart [14]. The first stage removes the failed skin tube and sutures adequately long and wide strips of oral mucosa on to the tunica albuginea of the corpora cavernosa. It takes 4–6 months for the revascularisation of the grafts to be stable. If a graft has revascularised (healed well), there is no contraction. During the second stage, the graft is re-tubularised to become the new urethra, covered by dartos subcutaneous tissue and the skin as a third layer (Figure 14.9b).

Another common cause of penile strictures is lichen sclerosus (balanitis xerotica obliterans, BXO), which can affect the penile urethral segment to a variable degree. The main disease process affects the fossa navicularis in most cases, giving rise to

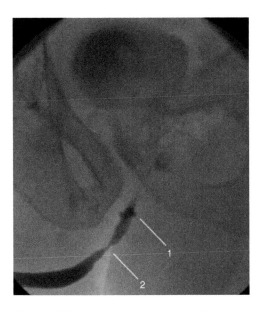

Figure 14.6 Postoperative urethrogram after pelvic fracture urethral reconstruction. The anastomotic site has as a typical diamond-shaped appearance (1). This patient developed a new ischemic mid-bulbar stricture (2) as a result of reduced spongiosal blood flow.

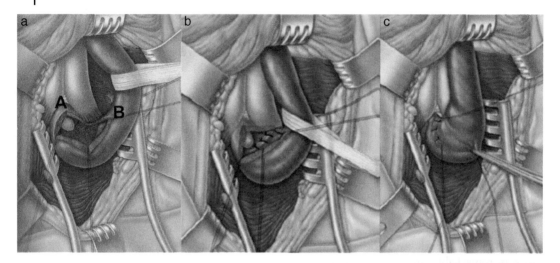

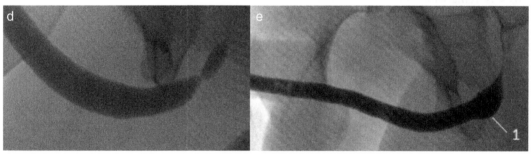

Figure 14.7 Short idiopathic bulbar stricture. In the non-transecting bulbar urethroplasty technique (NTABU), the superficial spongiofibrosis excised (a) and urethral plate reconstituted by mucosa–mucosa anastomosis (b). (c) The dorsal stricturotomy closed transversely. (d,e) Pre- and postoperative appearance after NTABU. Note the typical appearance of a 'bulge' on the ventral aspect of the bulbar urethra (e, 1) which is caused by buckling of the corpus spongiosum. Source: Bugeja *et al.* 2015 [12]. Reproduced with permission of AME Publishing Company.

a dense stricture with bladder outflow obstruction for many years, leading to over-distension of the upstream penile and bulbar urethra with every void. Urothelial damage leads to urinary extravasation and inflammation causing partial spongiofibrosis of the penile urethra to a variable degree (Figure 14.10). The penile urethra is more vulnerable than the bulbar urethral segment because the corpus spongiosum there is much thinner.

The latest urethroplasty techniques allow these challenging cases to be managed in a single stage [15], where two sublingual grafts quilted dorsally usually augment the affected urethral segments (Figure 10a), using an additional buccal mucosal graft for fossa navicularis reconstruction.

Use of Ultrasound in Urethroplasty Follow-up

Urethral sono-urethrography (SUG) was pioneered by McAninch in 1988 [16]. A high frequency linear probe (7–15 MHz) is used with the urethra gently distended with saline to evaluate stricture location, length and diameter. Even though retrograde urethrography (RUG) is more widely used, SUG is gaining popularity as an adjunctive diagnostic tool for urethral strictures, particularly in the bulbar urethra where it has been shown to be more sensitive than RUG in determining stricture length and location [17]. However, SUG is less sensitive for evaluation of posterior urethral strictures [18].

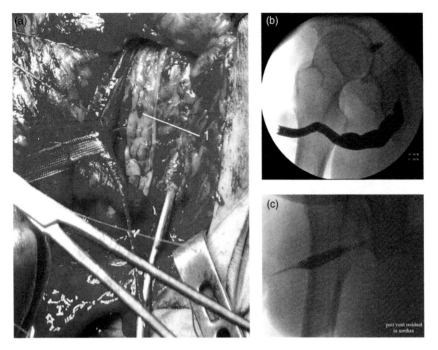

Figure 14.8 Long idiopathic bulbar stricture: (a) dorsal patch bulbar urethroplasty using oral mucosal graft (1). (b) Ascending urethrogram showing the dorsal patch of graft as a smooth irregular area producing a patent, if slightly wider, bulbar urethral segment. (c) Pooling of contrast in the augmented bulbar segment on voiding study accounting for post-micturition dribble.

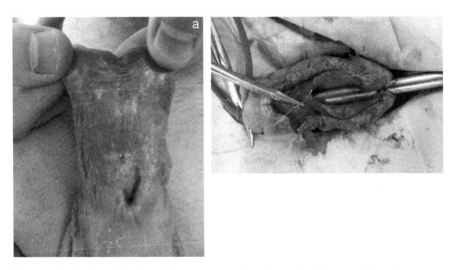

Figure 14.9 Penile urethroplasty. Two-stage procedure for proximal hypospadias stricture reconstruction. (a) Appearance of a healthy, good calibre urethral plate reconstructed with two sublingual grafts at the 'first stage' of the urethral reconstruction. (b) Three-layered neo-urethral retubularisation (graft, dartos, skin) at the 'second stage'.

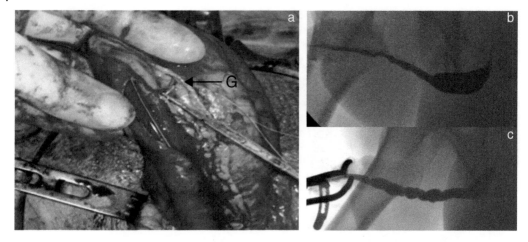

Figure 14.10 Full-length lichen sclerosus (BXO) stricture managed with a double sublingual dorsal augmentation technique. The urethra is mobilised from one side and opened dorsally. (a) The graft (G) is fixed dorsally to the tunica albuginea of the corpora cavernosa and then sewn to the urethral edges. (b) Pre- and (c) postoperative urethrograms.

SUG is the best investigation to determine the thickness of spongiofibrosis (areas of hyperechogenicity) and peri-urethral involvement (Figure 14.11), which in turn determines the choice of urethroplasty procedure [19]. From clinical experience we know that the relative thickness of spongiofibrosis in idiopathic bulbar strictures is minimal when compared with the bulk of healthy spongiosum, and that where spongiofibrosis affects the urethra circumferentially, subsequent tightening of the urethral lumen over time can occur.

The role of SUG as a screening tool for recurrent stricture after urethroplasty remains to be determined, being included in only 8% of follow-up protocols [4]. Stricture length or whether more than one urethral segment is affected by the disease process are still best evaluated by standard ascending and descending urethrogram.

Follow-up After Urethroplasty

Patients are followed-up after urethroplasty in order to assess outcome (success or failure) and detect recurrent strictures at an early stage. There is ongoing controversy as to which is the best modality [20]. Indeed, there is not even consensus as to what constitutes success or what defines a recurrent stricture [21]. Consequently, a 'successful' outcome, measured on clinical parameters alone, such as non-invasive flow rate [22] and patient reported outcome measure questionnaires (PROMs) [23], does not always equate to being stricture-free as patients clinically would not notice a recurrent stricture unless the calibre is less than 10 Fr [24].

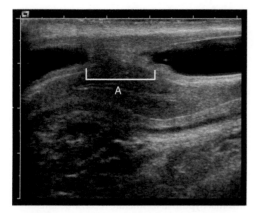

Figure 14.11 Ultrasound urethrogram of a stricture (A) at the penoscrotal junction appearing as an area of poor distendibility. The full cross-section of the urethral wall is visible, giving an indication of the spongiofibrosis extending into the underlying spongiosum.

Table 14.1 Follow-up protocol for urethroplasty.

Timescale	Procedure
2–3 weeks	Pericatheter urethrogram and removal of catheter
3 months	Urethrogram
	Flow rate, ultrasound PVR
	PROMs
1 year	Flow rate, ultrasound PVR
	PROMs
5 years	Urethrogram
	Flow rate, ultrasound PVR
	PROMs

PROMs, patient reported outcome measure questionnaires; PVR, post-void residual.

More objective postoperative investigations include urethrography [20] or endoscopy [25]. Stricture recurrence usually occurs within the first 2 years after urethroplasty [26] and therefore our follow-up is most intense during this period (Table 14.1). However, a further urethrogram is organised 5 years after urethroplasty because delayed stricture recurrence has been documented [27]. The old favourite of self-dilatation has been shown to be ineffective in preventing recurrence [28].

Radiological Appearance and Surgical Management of Recurrent Strictures After Urethroplasty

Patients who develop a recurrent stricture after urethroplasty usually present with recurring poor flow, recurrent urinary tract infections or, sometimes, haematuria. This can happen early (a few months after surgery) or after several years. We usually pick up potential problems at the 3-month follow-up urethrogram, where the first signs

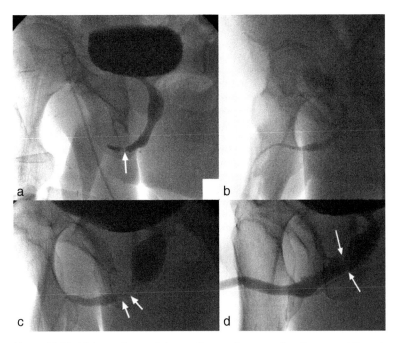

Figure 14.12 (a) Ascending and descending urethrogram showing near obliterative mid-bulbar stricture with pre-stenotic dilatation (arrow). (b) Descending urethrogram showing slight irregularity of the anastomotic site but no pre-stenotic dilatation and minimal post-void residual. (c) Subsequent descending study showing a longer bulbar stricture proximal to the site of anastomotic repair (arrows). (d) Typical appearance post-dorsal patch augmentation bulbar urethroplasty. Note that what appears to be a recurrent stricture (arrows) is in fact the proximal anastomosis of the graft to normal urethra and is only a 'relative' narrowing because the grafted segment is 'wider than normal' and is not flow-limiting.

of a suboptimal surgical outcome are usually apparent.

Generally, patients would be re-assessed by flow rate, post-void residual ultrasound and ascending and descending urethrogram to assess whether the problem is at the site of surgery or whether a stricture has developed in a different urethral segment. Most patients would then be evaluated cystoscopically at which time a urethral dilatation is performed (using serial plastic dilators over a safety guide wire). For early recurrent stricture, redo-urethroplasty is offered if feasible.

The choice of surgical technique depends on the underlying aetiology of the stricture and previous urethroplasty technique used, and is individual. A redo anastomotic repair is often inappropriate because of the risk of shortening of the urethra causing chordee.

A patient with a recurrent stricture is shown in Figure 14.12. He sustained a fall-astride bulbar crush injury when he was 12 years old. He did not receive any treatment at the time and continued to void with an obstructed flow into early adulthood, when he finally presented with acute urinary retention and a suprapubic catheter was inserted. Pre-operative urethrogram shows the obliterative stricture segment (Figure 14.12a), which was excised with an anastomotic repair technique. The 3-month postoperative follow-up urethrogram showed a slight irregularity at the anastomosis (Figure 14.12b), but he voided with an unobstructed flow.

At 5 years after surgery his flow deteriorated and a recurrent stricture was found on urethrogram (Figure 14.12c); a 1-cm stricture proximal to the previous anastomosis. This was surgically managed with a dorsal buccal graft augmentation bulbar urethroplasty technique with a good outcome (Figure 14.12d), albeit with some expected post-micturition dribble from the graft.

References

1 Wong S, Aboumarzouk O, Narahari R, O'Riordan A, Pickard, R. Simple urethral dilatation, endoscopic urethrotomy, and urethroplasty for urethral stricture disease in adult men. *Cochrane Database Syst Rev.* 2012; 12: CD006934.

2 Steenkamp JW, Heyns CF, de Kock ML. Internal urethrotomy versus dilation as treatment for male urethral strictures: a prospective, randomized comparison. *J Urol.* 1997; 157(1): 98–101.

3 Greenwell TJ, Castle C, Andrich DE, MacDonald JT, Nicol DL, Mundy AR. Repeat urethrotomy and dilation for the treatment of urethral stricture are neither clinically effective nor cost-effective. *J Urol.* 2004; 172(1): 275–277.

4 Meeks JJ, Erickson BA, Granieri MA, Gonzalez CM. Stricture recurrence after urethroplasty: a systematic review. *J Urol.* 2009; 182(4): 1266–1270.

5 Solanki S, Hussain S, Sharma DB, Solanki FS, Sharma D. Evaluation of healing at urethral anastomotic site by pericatheter retrograde urethrogram in patients with urethral stricture. *Urol Ann.* 2014; 6(4): 325–327.

6 Knoll L, Furlow W, Karsburg W. Pericatheter retrograde urethrography: introduction of a new device and technique. *J Urol.* 1989; 142(6): 1533–1535.

7 Pansadoro V, Emiliozzi P, Gaffi M, Scarpone P, DePaula F, Pizzo M. Buccal mucosa urethroplasty in the treatment of bulbar urethral strictures. *Urology.* 2003; 61(5): 1008–1010.

8 Heinke T, Gerharz EW, Bonfig R, Riedmiller H. Ventral onlay urethroplasty using buccal mucosa for complex stricture repair. *Urology* 2003; 61(5): 1004–1007.

9 Andrich DE, Mundy AR. What is the best technique for urethroplasty? *Eur Urol.* 2008; 54(5): 1031–1041.

10 Mundy AR. Anastomotic urethroplasty. *BJU Int*. 2005; 96(6): 921–944.

11 Andrich DE, Mundy AR. Non-transecting anastomotic bulbar urethroplasty: a preliminary report. *BJU Int*. 2012; 109(7): 1090–1094.

12 Bugeja S, Andrich DE, Mundy AR. Non-transecting bulbar urethroplasty. *Transl Androl Urol*. 2015; 4(1): 41–50.

13 Barbagli G, Palminteri E, Guazzoni G, Montorsi F, Turini D, Lazzeri M. Bulbar urethroplasty using buccal mucosa grafts placed on the ventral, dorsal or lateral surface of the urethra: are results affected by the surgical technique? *J Urol*. 2005; 174(3): 955–957; discussion 957–958.

14 Braka A. Hypospadias repair : the two-stage alternative. *BJU Int*. 1995; 76(Suppl 3): 31–41.

15 Tabassi K, Mansourian E, Yarmohamadi A. One-stage transperineal repair of pan-urethral stricture with dorsally placed buccal mucosal grafts. *J Urol*. 2011; 8(4): 307–312.

16 McAninch JW, Laing F, Jeffrey R. Sonourethrography in the evaluation of urethral strictures: a preliminary report. *J Urol*. 1988; 139(2): 294–297.

17 Morey AF, Mcaninch JW. Role of preoperative sonourethrography in bulbar urethral reconstruction. *J Urol*. 1997; 158(4): 1376–1379.

18 Ravikumar BR, Tejus C, Madappa KM, Prashant D, Dhayanand GS. A comparative study of ascending urethrogram and sono-urethrogram in the evaluation of stricture urethra. *Int Braz J Urol*. 2015; 41(2): 388–392.

19 Buckley JC, Wu AK, McAninch JW. Impact of urethral ultrasonography on decision-making in anterior urethroplasty. *BJU Int*. 2012; 109(3): 438–442.

20 Chapple C, Andrich DE, Atala, A, *et al*. SIU/ICUD Consultation on urethral strictures: the management of anterior urethral stricture disease using substitution urethroplasty. *Urology*. 2014; 83(3 Suppl), S31–47.

21 Choudhary S, Singh P, Sundar E, Kumar S, Sahai A. A comparison of sonourethrography and retrograde urethrography in evaluation of anterior urethral strictures. *Clin Radiol*. 2004; 59(8): 736–742.

22 Erickson BA, Breyer BN, McAninch JW. The use of uroflowmetry to diagnose recurrent stricture after urethral reconstructive surgery. *J Urol*. 2010; 184(4): 1386–1390.

23 Jackson MJ, Chaudhury I, Mangera A, *et al*. A prospective patient-centred evaluation of urethroplasty for anterior urethral stricture using a validated patient-reported outcome measure. *Eur Urol*. 2013; 64: 777–782.

24 Smith J. Urethral resistance to micturition. *Br J Urol*. 1968; 40(2): 125–56.

25 Goonesinghe SK, Hillary CJ, Nicholson TR, Osman NI, Chapple CR. Flexible cystourethroscopy in the follow-up of posturethroplasty patients and characterisation of recurrences. *Eur Urol*. 2015; 68(3): 523–529.

26 Yeung LL, Brandes SB. Urethroplasty practice and surveillance patterns: a survey of reconstructive urologists. *Urology*. 2013; 82(2): 471–475.

27 Andrich DE, Dunglison N, Greenwell TJ, Mundy AR. The long-term results of urethroplasty. *J Urol*. 2003; 170(1): 90–92.

28 Greenwell TJ, Castle C, Nicol DL. Clean intermittent self-catheterization does not appear to be effective in the prevention of urethral stricture recurrence. *Scand J Urol*. 2016; 50(1): 71–73.

15

The Postoperative Appearance and Follow-up of Urinary Tract Prostheses

Alex Kirkham

Introduction

The main purpose of this chapter is to address the postoperative appearances of two classes of device: artificial urinary sphincters and penile prostheses. We also describe the appearance of different forms of metallic stent. Some of the problems with these devices are common (in particular, infection); others are unique to the location. The indications for implantation, and the method for doing so, are beyond the scope of this chapter, and are described in detail elsewhere [1–4]. In addition, we focus on normal postoperative appearances and the ability of imaging to confirm a malfunctioning implant or diagnose the nature of the dysfunction. In most cases, routine imaging follow-up is not required when these prostheses are functioning well.

Penile Prostheses

Normal Appearance and Imaging Techniques

The types of penile prosthesis can be classified according to the number of components. The simplest is probably a variety of *malleable* implants, with only corporal components that can be varied in angulation, rather than length (e.g. Spectra, AMS/Boston Scientific, Marlborough, MA,

USA and Genesis, Coloplast, Fredensborg, Denmark).

Two-component devices are usually used when placement of a separate reservoir component would be technically challenging, and use a scrotal *resipump* to cycle fluid in and out of the inflatable corporal components of the device; the current available device has excellent mechanical reliability at the expense of incomplete flaccidity (AMS Ambicor) [5].

Two current three-piece devices are marketed: the Coloplast Titan and AMS Series 700. Both consist of a *reservoir* component (usually implanted in the space of Retzius, but sometimes deep to any of the muscle layers of the abdominal wall [1]), a *pump* component (almost always implanted into the scrotum, with connecting tubing passing next to or within the inguinal canal) and corporal components which consist of rigid and inflatable *corporal* parts (both of which can be varied in size).

Malleable implants are seen on plain radiography, as are parts of the corporal and pump components of inflated systems (Figure 15.1). However, most systems are now filled with saline rather than contrast (different from the usual practice with artificial sphincters) and plain films cannot be used to assess filling of the system, and certainly not the finer points of corporal positioning [6].

Radiology and Follow-up of Urologic Surgery, First Edition. Edited by Christopher Woodhouse and Alex Kirkham.
© 2018 John Wiley & Sons Ltd. Published 2018 by John Wiley & Sons Ltd.

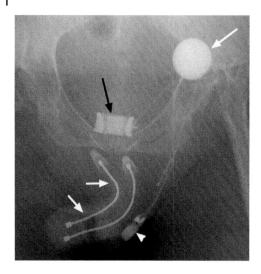

Figure 15.1 Plain film showing a malleable penile implant (white arrows), together with an artificial urinary sphincter with the cuff (black arrow) positioned at bladder neck, reservoir (long white arrow) in left iliac fossa and pump (arrowhead) in scrotum.

Both malleable and inflatable implants are clearly seen on both ultrasound (US; Figure 15.2) and magnetic resonance imaging (MRI; Figure 15.3). For the latter, the penis is usually scanned with the implant inflated and in the anatomical position.

The protocol should include at a minimum T2 sequences with 3-mm slices and an in plane resolution of 1 mm, together with at least one short T1 inversion recovery (STIR) sequence to detect fluid and inflammation. The routine use of T1 sequences and enhancement with gadolinium are not necessary [7]. All current devices are safe for MRI scanning, with the exception of the AMS Spectra, which shows heating of 1.6° in a 3T MRI (of limited clinical significance) [8]. Although fibrosis may complicate the picture, MRI almost always shows the tunica albuginea of the corpora cavernosa well [7].

Computerised tomography (CT) is of considerably lower resolution and is not routinely used for imaging the penis [7], but US shows the tunica albuginea of the corpora cavernosa well and the scrotum at high resolution. It also shows the edge of a malleable implant well, but has some important limitations. In a post-implant penis defining the margins of the tunica albuginea on US can be challenging, and deflated, deep or displaced reservoir balloons can be difficult to see. Overall, US is an excellent way to check for fluid in the system [9], but only MRI has

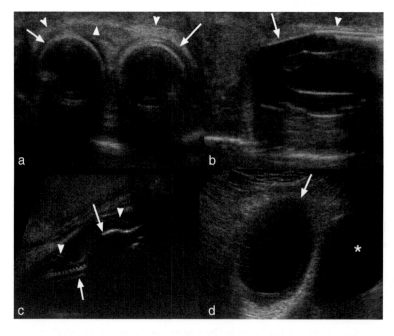

Figure 15.2 Ultrasound (US) of an inflatable penile prosthesis. (a,b) Axial and longitudinal images of the corporal component (arrows) with the device inflated; the echogenic tunica albuginea and Buck's fascia layer is shown by the arrowheads. (c) The pump (arrows), in this case surrounded by some fluid with fine strands (later shown to be infected). (d) The reservoir balloon (arrow) next to the bladder (asterisk).

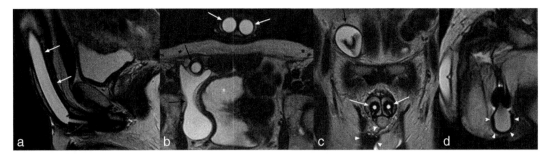

Figure 15.3 magnetic resonance imaging (MRI) appearance of a penile prosthesis on T2 sequences: (a,d) sagittal; (b) axial; and (c) coronal. The white arrow shows the inflated corporal components, black arrow the reservoir balloon and arrowheads the pump.

been shown to be accurate in the diagnosis of mechanical dysfunction [6, 10].

Problems of Positioning and Length

The position of all penile prostheses is well shown on MRI, and inflatable devices should by default be scanned inflated. Even in the case of severe intracavernosal fibrosis, the margins of the corpora cavernosa are of low signal on T2 sequences. Problems with positioning of the corporal components may occur either at implantation (in particular, crossover or perforation during placement) or at any time after implantation (in particular a breach of the corpora cavernosa in the crural part, or distal erosion, occurring in around 1%, although in some series up to 6.5%) [1, 11]. In general, these are well seen on MRI, although the spatial resolution is not accurate enough to characterise impending erosion. The 'supersonic transporter deformity' (Figure 15.4), caused by a hypermobile, non-tumescent glans, is often a result of a slightly proximal position of the corporal component, with failure to lie against the tips. The diagnosis is often apparent clinically [12], although it may sometimes be useful to show the position of these components on MRI. Overall, US may allow a more dynamic examination with the device inflated, although there is no published description of its utility.

As well as becoming displaced, implants may rarely show aneurysmal dilatation (Figure 15.5) or rupture (a common mode of failure in devices implanted for >10 years).

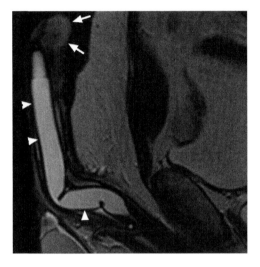

Figure 15.4 Sagittal T2 image of a slightly oversized penile prosthesis (arrowheads show the corporal component), with some mild buckling at the base. This appearance can be produced by positioning for the scan, with dorsal downwards pressure producing a 'kink', but in this image it is a little more conspicuous than normal. The tip also shows a 'floppy glans' or 'supersonic transporter' deformity (arrows) – sometimes occurring when the prosthesis is too short but often, as in this case, in spite of snug fitting of the corporal component against cavernosal tips.

Both are apparent on MRI – with the latter demonstrated by incompletely inflated cylinders with the device inflated, or an incompletely distended reservoir when it is not.

Penile shortening is commonly reported with inflatable implants, and there is some evidence that it can be mitigated by early

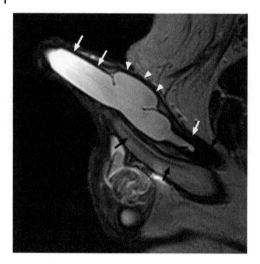

Figure 15.5 Sagittal T2 image of aneurysmal dilatation in a penile prosthesis. The white arrows show the inflated corporal component, and the arrowheads the aneurysmal part. Black arrows show the urethra.

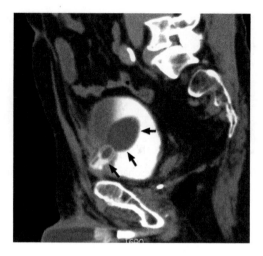

Figure 15.6 Sagittal image from a CT urogram showing erosion of the reservoir balloon (arrows) into the bladder. The patient had only irritative bladder symptoms.

inflation [13] or by a slight over-sizing of the corporal components [14]. The danger of the latter is of pain on inflation and deformity from 'kinking' or 'buckling' of the cavernosal components, a diagnosis that may be difficult clinically but is usually apparent on MRI (Figure 15.4) [11]. However, such kinking may be becoming rarer with early inflation protocols and improved cylinder design [15].

The reservoir balloon is well seen within the abdomen on both CT and MRI (and in most cases on US), and although displacement is rare, erosion into bladder or rectum has been reported (Figure 15.6).

Modern penile prostheses are coated with either antibiotic-impregnated compounds or a hydrophilic layer that can be dipped in and retain antibiotics at operation, with good evidence that such a strategy has been effective [16]; the current rate of infections of penile prostheses over their lifetimes is 0.5–3.5% [1, 17]. Infections occur spontaneously or as the result of erosion to the outside, and are discussed in detail together with infections in artificial urinary sphincters.

Artificial Urinary Sphincters

By far the most common artificial urinary sphincter device is the AMS800 (American Medical Systems/Boston Scientific, Marlborough, MA, USA), which may have been implanted in over 100 000 men since its introduction in 1972 [18]. Although the most common location for implantation is in the bulbar urethra in men [19, 20], it can also be implanted around the bladder neck in men [21] and in women [22]. Alternatives, such as the Zephyr [23] and Flowsecure [23] devices, have attempted to address some of the deficiencies of the established device, but there are currently few data concerning their efficacy [24].

Although there is some benefit in using double cuffs in patients with severe incontinence [25], the most common configuration is with a single cuff, a scrotal or labial pump and a balloon in an extraperitoneal intra-abdominal plane. The AMS800 may be filled with saline or, more commonly, isotonic radiographic contrast, so that plain film radiography often shows filling of each of the components well (Figure 15.1), although it is less effective at showing their relation to soft tissues. Adequate filling, together with normal cycling on compressing the scrotal component, are usually adequate to confirm normal mechanical operation.

Disorders of Function and Position

A malfunctioning artificial urinary sphincter (AUS) may be a result of misplacement or displacement, rupture, erosion, infection and in some cases the inherent limitations of the device. The last is important because two critical choices are made at the time of implantation: the size of the cuff and the pressure in the reservoir balloon, which determines the pressure in the whole system. It is not known what proportion of erosions are caused by later pressure necrosis [26], but is likely to be related to the pressure in the system. For the cuff, too large and the urethral closure pressure may fall below the pressure of around 50 cm water that is usually associated with adequate continence [27, 28]; too small and catheterisation or cystoscopy become more hazardous [19].

US and MRI, with parameters similar to those used for penile prostheses [29], may be used to show the components of the artificial sphincter (Figures 15.7 and 15.8). As in the case of penile prostheses, the ability of MRI to accurately define the relation of the components to important structures (in particular the urethra) is unrivalled: it will show an 'unwrapped' or twisted cuff (Figure 15.9) and misplacement in bulbar urethra or bladder neck. There is an overlap here with fluoroscopy, which may be used to confirm the clinical suspicion of erosion (Figure 15.10), and can demonstrate the relationship of the cuff to the urethral lumen.

Although erosion is a serious complication, more common is a degree of incontinence with a correctly implanted device. This is often investigated with urodynamics to confirm that the cause is not bladder overactivity, but ultimately the most useful information is the pressure that is being exerted on the urethral lumen by the cuff, which can be reduced because of a fibrous capsule [30]

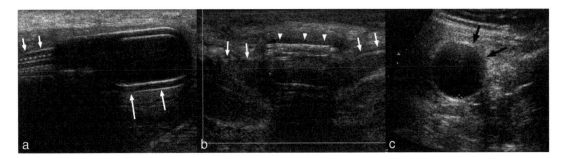

Figure 15.7 The appearance of the artificial urinary sphincter (AUS) on US: (a) the pump, (b) a bulbar cuff, and (c) the reservoir balloon.

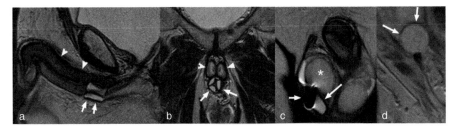

Figure 15.8 An artificial urinary sphincter on MRI: (a,b) sagittal and coronal T2-weighted images of a bulbar cuff (the arrowheads show the corpora cavernosa), (c) the pump lying adjacent to the right testis (asterisk) and (d) the reservoir balloon.

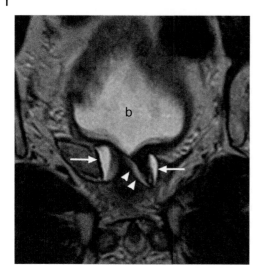

Figure 15.9 Sagittal T2 image showing an AUS cuff appropriately positioned at the bladder neck (arrows). However, there is a 180° twist (requiring operative correction) in the cuff, shown by the arrowheads. b, bladder.

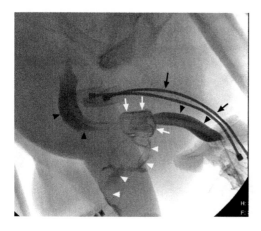

Figure 15.10 Retrograde urethrogram showing contrast in the urethra (black arrow heads) and around the AUS cuff (white arrows), with a fistulous track extending to skin (white arrowheads). A malleable penile prosthesis is also seen (black arrows); note that no contrast is seen around it.

or a variety of mechanical problems. Urethral pressure profilometry has been used to measure this pressure [27] but inherently involves withdrawing a catheter through a closed AUS cuff. Probably better is the technique of retrograde urethral pressure measurement, the pressure at which contrast passes the cuff on retrograde instillation (Figure 15.11) [31].

Infection in Implanted Devices

Almost all models of penile prosthesis [32] and artificial sphincter [1] incorporate systems for antibiotic coating which have significantly reduced infection rates. Nevertheless, it is still one of the main reasons for failure of artificial urinary sphincters, with erosion or infection occurring in 8% in a recent series [28]. Infections vary in timing: from acute, purulent cases occurring weeks after implantation to more chronic presentations with pain, in particular in those caused by coagulase-negative staphylococci [32]. In both types of implant, a biofilm containing bacteria can be identified in a significant proportion of patients whose devices are removed for other reasons [33]. The role of imaging in infection is uncertain: if severe (presenting with pain, redness or fluctuance over sphincter components), it is likely to be apparent clinically [32]. Imaging with MRI and US may show fluid around the components, inflammation (in particular on MRI) and tenderness to pressure over the components (on US), and may be useful for surgical planning, but fluid does not necessarily equate to infection: some fluid may be seen around uninfected implants, as well as a fibrous pseudocapsule (Figure 15.12). On MRI, the presence of inflammatory change, in particular high signal oedema on STIR and enhancement after MR contrast (Figure 15.12) [7], may be more specific, and for this reason MRI may be preferable to US, which can delineate fluid but may be less sensitive for inflammatory change. In more indolent infections where the diagnosis is more challenging, the imaging appearances are often equivocal: with less inflammation it can be challenging to determine whether fluid around an implant is infected. There are no published data on the accuracy of imaging for the diagnosis of infected urinary

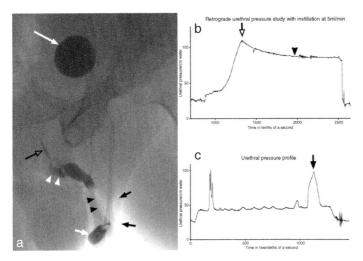

Figure 15.11 (a) Method of retrograde urethral pressure study: after placement of a 6 Fr catheter into the proximal penile urethra, a cuff (black arrows) is placed around the distal penis and inflated to 100 cm water, and contrast instilled at 5 mL/min. The point at which contrast passes the AUS cuff (indicated by the black open arrow) usually coincides with the peak in the pressure trace seen in (b) (black open arrow). The absolute pressure exerted by the cuff is measured with reference to the pressure at the level of the symphysis (measured after the catheter is withdrawn). With an AUS the peak pressure reaches a plateau (black arrowhead in b), and this plateau probably more accurately reflects the pressure exerted by the cuff. A urethral pressure profile can also be obtained, but involves catheterisation through the cuff: the pressure exerted by the cuff in the same patient is represented by the peak (c, black arrow).

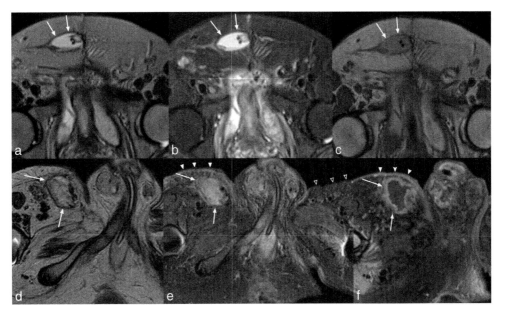

Figure 15.12 Fluid around the tubing of an artificial urinary sphincter on MRI in two scenarios. (a–c) Postoperative haematoma and serous fluid is seen around the tubing: note that on the T2 axial sequence (a) the margin of the fluid is well-defined, and on STIR (b) there is little surrounding oedema. (c) The T1-weighted sequence shows high signal consistent with blood. (d–f) The fluid is from an infection (proven at explantation). On T2 (d) the contents are a little heterogeneous, and on STIR (e) there is oedema around the fluid and in the adjacent skin (arrowheads) – different from the other side (outline arrowheads). (f) Prominent, slightly irregular enhancement around the fluid (arrows) and adjacent skin (arrowheads).

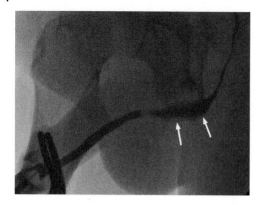

Figure 15.13 Urethrogram showing a widely patent Urolume stent (arrows) in the bulbar urethra.

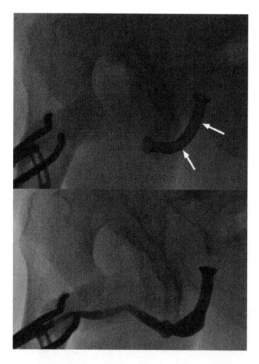

Figure 15.14 Plain film and urethrogram images of a Memokath stent (arrows) in the membranous and bulbar urethra.

tract implants. We have found that although it may help the surgical approach by localising pockets of fluid, it only rarely changes the clinical impression of the presence of significant infection.

Finally, where infection in an artificial urinary sphincter is caused by erosion of the cuff component, urethrogram is a straightforward way of confirming the diagnosis (Figure 15.10).

Metallic Stents

The Urolume (American Medical Systems) metallic wall stent has been used for the treatment of recurrent bulbar urethral stricture disease, benign prostatic hyperplasia (BPH) and detrusor external sphincter dyssynergia [34], as well as obstruction after prostate cancer surgery [3]. Although there is debate about its efficacy [3], it has not been available since 2012, predominantly because of problems with pain, migration and re-occlusion [35]. The stents are well seen on fluoroscopy, which is likely to be the best modality for assessing position and luminal calibre (Figure 15.13).

Although not currently available in the USA, thermo-expandable metallic stents (in particular, Memokath; PNN Medical, Denmark) can be used in both the urethra (Figure 15.14) and ureter. Although encrustation and migration do occur, removal is usually straightforward and rarely results in stricturing. The stents are well seen on plain radiographs and at fluoroscopy, which is often used to demonstrate patency. Their position is also well shown on CT.

References

1 Trost L, Wanzek P, Bailey G. A practical overview of considerations for penile prosthesis placement. *Nat Rev Urol.* 2015; 13(1): 33–46.

2 Amend B, Toomey P, Sievert K-D. Artificial sphincter. *Curr Opin Urol.* 2013; 23(6): 520–527.

3 McNamara ER, Webster GD, Peterson AC. The UroLume stent revisited: the Duke experience. *Urology*. 2013; 82(4): 933–936.

4 Mehta SS, Tophill PR. Memokath® stents for the treatment of detrusor sphincter dyssynergia (DSD) in men with spinal cord injury: The Princess Royal Spinal Injuries Unit 10-year experience. *Spinal Cord*. 2005; 44(1): 1–6.

5 Lux M, Reyes-Vallejo L, Morgentaler A, Levine LA. Outcomes and satisfaction rates for the redesigned 2-piece penile prosthesis. *J Urol*. 2007; 177(1): 262–266.

6 Moncada I, Jara J, Cabello R, Monzo J, Hernández C. Radiological assessment of penile prosthesis: the role of magnetic resonance imaging. *World J Urol*. 2004; 22(5): 371–377.

7 Kirkham AP, Illing R, Minhas S, Minhas S, Allen C. MR imaging of nonmalignant penile lesions. *Radiographics*. 2008; 28(3): 837–853.

8 Lowe G, Smith RP, Costabile RA. A catalog of magnetic resonance imaging compatibility of penile prostheses. *J Sex Med*. 2012; 9(5): 1482–1487.

9 Suarez G, Baum N. Ultrasonography in evaluation of mechanical problems of inflatable penile prosthesis. *Urology*. 1987; 30(4): 388–389.

10 Moncada I, Hernández C, Jara J, *et al.* Buckling of cylinders may cause prolonged penile pain after prosthesis implantation: a case control study using magnetic resonance imaging of the penis. *J Urol*. 1998; 160(1): 67–71.

11 Carson CC, Mulcahy JJ, Govier FE. Efficacy, safety and patient satisfaction outcomes of the AMS 700CX inflatable penile prosthesis: results of a long-term multicenter study. AMS 700CX Study Group. *J Urol*. 2000; 164(2): 376–380.

12 Mulhall JP, Kim FJ. Reconstructing penile supersonic transporter (SST) deformity using glanulopexy (glans fixation). *Urology*. 2001; 57(6): 1160–1162.

13 Caraceni E, Utizi L, Angelozzi G. Pseudo-capsule 'coffin effect': how to

prevent penile retraction after implant of three-piece inflatable prosthesis. *Arch Ital Urol Androl*. 2014; 86(2): 135–137.

14 Henry GD, Carrion R, Jennermann C, Wang R. Prospective evaluation of postoperative penile rehabilitation: penile length/girth maintenance 1 year following Coloplast Titan inflatable penile prosthesis. *J Sex Med*. 2015; 12(5): 1298–1304.

15 Hakky TS, Wang R, Henry GD. The evolution of the inflatable penile prosthetic device and surgical innovations with anatomical considerations. *Curr Urol Rep*. 2014; 15(6): 410.

16 Serefoglu EC, Mandava SH, Gokce A, Chouhan JD, Wilson SK, Hellstrom WJ. Long-term revision rate due to infection in hydrophilic-coated inflatable penile prostheses: 11-year follow-up. *J Sex Med*. 2012; 9(8): 2182–2186.

17 Henry GD, Wilson SK. Updates in inflatable penile prostheses. *Urol Clin North Am*. 2007; 34(4): 535–547, vi.

18 Lucas MG, Bosch RJ, Burkhard FC, *et al.* EAU guidelines on surgical treatment of urinary incontinence. *Eur Urol*. 2012; 62(6): 1118–1129.

19 Andrich DE, Mundy AR. Urethral reconstruction and artificial urinary sphincters. In Muneer A, Arya M, Jordan G (eds). *Atlas of Male Genitourethral Surgery: The Illustrated Guide*. John Wiley & Sons, Ltd, Chichester. 2014: 117–133.

20 Phé V, Rouprêt M, Mozer P, Chartier-Kastler E. Trends in the landscape of artificial urinary sphincter implantation in men and women in France over the past decade. *Eur Urol*. 2013; 63(2): 407–408.

21 Hoy NY, Rourke KF. Artificial urinary sphincter outcomes in the 'fragile urethra'. *Urology*. 2015; 86(3): 618–624.

22 Costa P, Poinas G, Ben Naoum K, *et al.* Long-term results of artificial urinary sphincter for women with type III stress urinary incontinence. *Eur Urol*. 2013; 63(4): 753–758.

23 Staerman F, G-Llorens C, Leon P, Leclerc Y. ZSI 375 artificial urinary sphincter

for male urinary incontinence: a preliminary study. *BJU Int*. 2013; 111(4 Pt B): E202–206.

24 Chung E, Ranaweera M, Cartmill R. Newer and novel artificial urinary sphincters (AUS): the development of alternatives to the current AUS device. *BJU Int*. 2012; 110(Suppl 4): 5–11.

25 O'Connor RC, Lyon MB, Guralnick ML, Bales GT. Long-term follow-up of single versus double cuff artificial urinary sphincter insertion for the treatment of severe postprostatectomy stress urinary incontinence. *Urology*. 2008; 71(1): 90–93.

26 Hussain M, Greenwell TJ, Venn SN, Mundy AR. The current role of the artificial urinary sphincter for the treatment of urinary incontinence. *J Urol*. 2005; 174(2): 418–424.

27 Chung E, Cartmill R. Diagnostic challenges in the evaluation of persistent or recurrent urinary incontinence after artificial urinary sphincter (AUS) implantation in patients after prostatectomy. *BJU Int*. 2013; 112: 32–35.

28 Linder BJ, Rivera ME, Ziegelmann MJ, Elliott DS. Long-term outcomes following artificial urinary sphincter placement: an analysis of 1082 cases at Mayo Clinic. *Urology*. 2015; 86(3): 602–607.

29 Deng J, Hall-Craggs MA, Craggs MD, *et al*. Three-dimensional MRI of the male urethrae with implanted artificial sphincters: initial results. *Br J Radiol*. 2006; 79(942): 455–463.

30 Bugeja S, Ivaz SL, Frost A, Andrich DE, Mundy AR. Urethral atrophy after implantation of an artificial urinary sphincter: fact or fiction? *BJU Int*. 2016; 117(4): 669–676.

31 Comiter CV, Sullivan MP, Yalla SV. Retrograde leak point pressure for evaluating postradical prostatectomy incontinence. *Urology*. 1997; 49(2): 231–236.

32 Muench PJ. Infections versus penile implants: the war on bugs. *J Urol*. 2013; 189(5): 1631–1637.

33 Hofer MD, Gonzalez CM. Current concepts in infections associated with penile prostheses and artificial sphincters. *Urol Clin North Am*. 2015; 42(4): 485–492.

34 Badlani GH, Press SM, Defalco A, Oesterling JE, Smith AD. Urolume endourethral prosthesis for the treatment of urethral stricture disease: long-term results of the North American Multicenter UroLume Trial. *Urology*. 1995; 45(5): 846–856.

35 Wilson TS, Lemack GE, Dmochowski RR. UroLume stents: lessons learned. *J Urol*. 2002; 167(6): 2477–2480.

Index

Note: Illustrations (figures and tables) are comprehensively referred to from the text. Therefore, significant items in illustrations have only been given a page reference in the absence of their concomitant mention in the text referring to that illustration.

Radiology and Follow-up of Urologic Surgery, First Edition. Edited by Christopher Woodhouse and Alex Kirkham.
© 2018 John Wiley & Sons Ltd. Published 2018 by John Wiley & Sons Ltd.

Printed and bound by CPI Group (UK) Ltd, Croydon, CR0 4YY

16/04/2025

14658552-0004